I0887763

Berakhyah Ben Natronai ha-Nakdan,
Sefer Ko'aḥ ha-Avanim
(*On the Virtue of the Stones*).
Hebrew Text and English Translation

Études sur le Judaïsme Médiéval

Fondées par

Georges Vajda

Dirigées par

Paul B. Fenton

TOME XL

Berakhyah Ben Natronai ha-Nakdan, *Sefer Ko'aḥ ha-Avanim* (*On the Virtue of the Stones*). Hebrew Text and English Translation

With a Lexicological Analysis of the Romance Terminology and Source Study

Edited, translated, and annotated by

Gerrit Bos and Julia Zwink

TUTA SUB AEGIDE PALLAS · 1683 ·

BRILL

LEIDEN • BOSTON
2010

This book is printed on acid-free paper.

Library of Congress Cataloging-in-Publication Data

Berechiah ben Natronai, ha-Nakdan, 12th/13th cent.
[Koah ha-avanim. English & Hebrew]
Sefer ko'ah ha-avanim = (On the virtue of the stones) / Berechiah ben Natronai ha-Nakdan ; Hebrew text and English translation with a Lexicological analysis of the Romance Terminology and Source Study ; edited, translated, and annotated by Gerrit Bos and Julia Zwink.
p. cm. – (Etudes sur le judaïsme médiéval, ISSN 0169-815X ; t. 40)
Includes bibliographical references and index.
ISBN 978-90-04-18310-0 (hard cover : alk. paper)
1. Gems–Folklore. 2. Medicine, Medieval–Folklore. 3. Magic. 4. Lapidaries (Medieval literature) 5. Berechiah ben Natronai, ha-Nakdan, 12th/13th cent. Sefer Ko'ah ha-avanim. I. Zwink, Julia. II. Bos, Gerrit, 1925- III. Title. IV. Series.

GR805.B47 2010
133'.25538–dc22

2010002321

ISSN: 0169-815X
ISBN: 978 90 04 18310 0

Copyright 2010 by Koninklijke Brill NV, Leiden, The Netherlands.
Koninklijke Brill NV incorporates the imprints Brill, Hotei Publishing, IDC Publishers, Martinus Nijhoff Publishers and VSP.

All rights reserved. No part of this publication may be reproduced, translated, stored in a retrieval system, or transmitted in any form or by any means, electronic, mechanical, photocopying, recording or otherwise, without prior written permission from the publisher.

Authorization to photocopy items for internal or personal use is granted by Koninklijke Brill NV provided that the appropriate fees are paid directly to The Copyright Clearance Center, 222 Rosewood Drive, Suite 910, Danvers, MA 01923, USA.
Fees are subject to change.

PRINTED IN THE NETHERLANDS

CONTENTS

PREFACE

I am grateful for the opportunity to present to the reader this edition and translation of the lapidary composed by Berakhyah Ben Natronai ha-Nakdan. The text of the lapidary features in the margin of a single liturgical manuscript and was copied by a scribe who hardly new any Hebrew and did not understand the text at all, so that it is replete with mistakes and corruptions. Recently, the text was published anonymously in an uncritical edition that is full of mistakes. Berakhyah's lapidary, allegedly the oldest Hebrew lapidary that has come down to us, received much attention in the past because it contains possibly one of the earliest references to the sailor's compass called "aimant". The book describes 72 stones which are arranged in alphabetical order as is common for lapidaries, with the exception of stones 68 to 70. The virtues of the stones are of a medical-scientific character and/or of a magical-supernatural one; we do not find any reference to allegorical or astrological connotations of the stones.

A major source consulted by Berakhyah for the composition of this treatise are the medieval French translations and adaptations of the lapidary entitled *De lapidibus* composed by Marbode of Rennes. These medieval French versions were composed in Anglo-Norman England. The version which Berakhyah consulted more than any other for the composition of his stonebook is the Cambridge Version of Marbode. The Cambridge Version was Berakhyah's main source for at least 43 of the 72 stones featuring in his lapidary, as is shown in the supplement in the detailed analysis by Julia Zwink.

Marbode's *De lapidibus* was translated twice into Hebrew: by an anonymous author under the title *Ellu shemot ha-avanim ha-ṭovim* and by Jacob ben Reuben in a verse translation entitled *Sefer ha-ʿOsher*. The anonymous translation is not derivative upon a Latin Marbode Vorlage but a French one, as it shares several old French terms with French versions of Marbode's Lapidary.

A table comparing the texts and translations of both versions and their analysis on the basis of the versions in Old French they drew upon (above all the Cambridge Version) would have been an ideal and ultimate presentation of the material at hand. Unfortunately such a presentation requiring years of intensive research and analysis was not possible within the context of the present project and the researchers involved. Of these researchers I am especially grateful to my colleague Gad Freudenthal. He has read with meticulous care all my transcriptions and translations, compared them with the text of the manuscript, corrected mistakes, and made suggestions for alternative, better readings. I am also thankful to my friend Eric Pellow who with his experience in reading Hebrew manuscripts and intimate knowledge of medieval Hebrew literature provided likely readings for some of the many corruptions featuring in the text. Finally I thank the Deutsche Forschungsgemeinschaft for their financial support of this project.

ABBREVIATIONS

General Abbreviations

Angl.-Nor.	Anglo-Norman
Arab.	Arabic
c.	century
Cat.	Catalan
cf.	confer; compare
ed.	editor
e.g.	exempli gratia; for example
et al.	et alii; and others
fol.	folio
Fr.	French
Gr.	(Ancient) Greek
Gr.-Lat.	Graeco-Latin
i.e.	id est; that is
id.	idem; the same
It.	Italian
Judeo-Fr.	Judeo-French
Lat.	Latin
loc. cit.	loco citato; in the place cited
M. Fr.	Middle French
M. Lat.	Medieval Latin
Mod. Fr.	Modern French
Ms.	manuscript
no.	number
O. Cat.	Old Catalan
O. Engl.	Old English
O. Fr.	Old French
O. It.	Old Italian
O. Occ.	Old Occitan
O. Port.	Old Portuguese
O. Sp.	Old Spanish
s.v.	sub voce; under the headword

Abbreviations and Symbols to the Edition and Translation

In Hebrew text

⟨...⟩	hiatus in the text
⟨אאא⟩	added by the editor
[...]	corrupt reading
A =	Anonymous Hebrew translation MS Bern
r =	Riddle, ed. Marbode

In translation

⟨...⟩	hiatus in the translation
[...]	added by the translator

INTRODUCTION[1]

1. *The Author*

Berakhyah Ben Natronai ha-Nakdan was a Hebrew scholar, punctuator, commentator of the Bible, and fabulist whose life and identity have been the object of much speculation in the past, as there is very little definite information. Especially in the nineteenth century his life and literary activities received much attention from Jewish scholars and promoters of the "Wissenschaft des Judentums," such as Julius Fürst, Leopold Zunz, Heinrich Graetz, and Moritz Steinschneider, next to other scholars like Adolph Neubauer, Henri Gross, and Joseph Jacobs. To quote just a few of the opinions held by these scholars: Graetz called him "a poor scribe, also called 'Crispia', flor. 1230–1245."[2] According to Jacobs, Berakhyah is identical with Benedictus le Puncteur of Oxford and was one of the most important English Jews who lived around 1190.[3] Steinschneider, in his catalogue of the Hebrew books in the Bodleian Library,[4] refers to him as a "punctator" (punctuator), "Gallus" (from France), also called "Crispia", and adds that if he is the interpreter or epitomizer of Sa'adya Ga'on's "Beliefs and Opinions", he must have flourished before 1170; in his *Die hebräischen Übersetzungen* he states that we do not know for certain Berakhyah's native country, that we do not have sufficient proof to suppose that it might have been England, and that he lived in the thirteenth

[1] I thank Susan Einbinder for her comments to an earlier version of the introduction.

[2] H. Graetz, *Geschichte der Juden von den ältesten Zeiten bis auf die Gegenwart. Aus den Quellen neu bearbeitet*. Bd. 7: *Geschichte der Juden von Maimunis Tod (1205) bis zur Verbannung der Juden aus Spanien und Portugal*. 4th revised edition, Leipzig n.d., p. 78.

[3] *Fables of Aesop*, London 1889. Jacobs' theory that Berakhyah was no one else but Benedictus le Puncteur (Benedict le Pointur) found support in C. Roth, *The Jews of Medieval Oxford*, Oxford 1951, pp. 117–118; and *A History of the Jews in England*, 3rd ed. Oxford 1964, pp. 126, 280, note k.

[4] M. Steinschneider, *Catalogus Librorum Hebraeorum in Bibliotheca Bodleiana*. Berlin 1852–1860. Repr. Hildesheim 1964, col. 796.

century,[5] and in his *Lapidarien* adds that he is of French origin.[6] Gross thought that he lived in Dreux, in the north of France and is identical with Crespia.[7]

The divergent opinions held by these scholars were, with the exception of Graetz, critically reviewed and summarized by Herman Gollancz in 1902 with the following words: "This, then, is in effect almost all that has been hitherto written concerning our author, and the result is comparatively unsatisfactory. Neither the date of his birth, nor of his activity, is fixed with any precision; the place whence he came, the amount of knowledge he possessed, the sources which he utilized, the whole character of his works, all these points have not yet been definitely determined."[8] Gollancz then unfolds his own theory concerning the author's life and works based on the few data we possess. From the rarity of the family name he surmises that he had a brother, a Tosaphist in France, called Samuel ha-Nakdan who is mentioned for the year 1175 and that he was not so much a punctuator of the Bible himself but hailed from a family of Nakdanim. He refutes the identification of Berakhyah with Crespia or Crispia ha-Nakdan, suggests that he was born early in the twelfth century in the Provence and may have moved at some time to the north of France, and that his literary activity reached its zenith between 1160 and 1170.[9] Gollancz's own theory concerning Berakhyah's identity was in its turn critically reviewed by Nathan Porges,[10] Jacob Gutman,[11] Israel Lévi,[12] and Steinschneider.[13] Especially Lévi was sharp in his critique of Gollancz's reconstruction of Berakhyah's biography when he concluded that "his attempt to freshen up the old hypothesis had failed".[14]

---

[5] M. Steinschneider, *Die hebräischen Übersetzungen im Mittelalter und die Juden als Dolmetscher*. Berlin 1893. Repr. Graz 1956, p. 961.

[6] M. Steinschneider, "Lapidarien, ein culturgeschichtlicher Versuch", in: *Semitic Studies in Memory of Alexander Kohut*, Berlin 1897. Repr. Jerusalem 1972, pp. 42–72, p. 62.

[7] H. Gross, *Gallia Judaica. Dictionnaire géographique de la France*. Paris 1897, pp. 180–181.

[8] H. Gollancz (ed.), *The Ethical Treatises of Berachya, Son of Rabbi Natronai ha-Nakdan being the Compendium and the Maṣref*. London 1902, pp. xi–xxii, esp. p. xxii.

[9] Ibid., pp. xxii–xxvii.

[10] in: *Zeitschrift für Hebraeische Bibliographie*, vol. 7.1, Frankfurt a.M. 1903, p. 36ff.

[11] in: *Monatschrift für Geschichte und Wissenschaft des Judentums*, vol. 46, p. 536f.

[12] in: *Revue des Études juives*, vol. 46 (1903), p. 285ff.

[13] in: *The Jewish Quarterly Review*, vol. 17 (1905), p. 581.

[14] *Revue des Études juives*, vol. 46 (1903), p. 288.

Following these discussions about the author's identity more than half a century would pass without any fundamental new insight into the question of the author's biography. Thus, Moses Hadas, the translator of Berakhyah's *Mishlei Shuʿalim* (Fox Fables) into English states that "there is very little information about the life of Rabbi Berakhyah ben Natronai ha-Nakdan", that he was "French, born perhaps in Burgundy, and that he spent much time in Provence", and that he is possibly identical with Benedictus le Puncteur.[15] And A.M. Habermann remarks in the entry on Berakhyah in the *Encyclopaedia Judaica*, published in 1971, that he lived at the end of the twelfth-thirteenth century, has been identified with Benedictus le Puncteur, and also with Crespia or Crispia which has proven to be wrong, that he lived in Normandy, and at some time also in England.[16]

In 1974 Norman Golb came up with new data concerning Berakhyah's biography and literary activity in his monograph on the history of the Jews of Rouen,[17] and in his history of the Jews in medieval Normandy published in 1998.[18] However, it seems that also his "biography" is not the final word on Berakhyah's life and activities, as it has been criticized by a number of scholars. According to Golb, Berakhyah lived in the second half of the twelfth century in the city of Radom (= Rouen) in Normandy which was at that time ruled by the Angevin kings of England whose rule is marked by generous liberties and protection granted to the Jews. This political situation facilitated the development of Rouen into a center of both religious and secular learning, with prominent scholars like Samuel Ben Meir (Rashbam), Eliezer of Beaugency, Abraham ibn Ezra and Berakhyah. While Samuel Ben Meir and Eliezer of Beaugency were concentrating as biblical commentators on the Jewish religious tradition, both Ibn Ezra and Berakhyah took great interest in secular science and wisdom from non-Jewish sources and played a central role in its transfer to the Jews in northwestern Europe. Ibn Ezra was above all active in promoting the introduction of popular and learned science, such as grammar, mathematics, astronomy and astrology derived from Arab sources

[15] M. Hadas, *Fables of a Jewish Aesop*. Translated from the Fox Fables of Berakhyah ha-Nakdan. New York & London 1967. p. ix.

[16] A.M. Habermann, entry "Berakhyah Ben Natronai ha-Nakdan," *Encyclopaedia Judaica*, vol. 4, 1971, cols. 596–598.

[17] N. Golb, *History and Culture of the Jews of Rouen in the Middle Ages* (in Hebrew) Tel Aviv 1976, pp. 120–144.

[18] N. Golb, *The Jews in medieval Normandy. A social and intellectual history*. Cambridge 1998, pp. 321–347.

into Jewish circles, his fellow citizen Berakhyah concentrated foremost on the transmission of science and wisdom to his Jewish compatriots derived from Christian sources.

2. *Literary Activity*

Berakhyah's literary activity should be seen in the light of the following confession in the work called by the editor Gollancz *Dodi we-Nekhdi* according to which he saw himself as a transmitter of foreign (Greek, Arabic) lore and literature, philosophy and science which were hidden in the works by Christian authors to his Jewish compatriots:

> I, Berachya, son of Natronai, was worried in thought till I girded my loins, and translated these subjects into Hebrew. I found them in non-Jewish writings, translated as they were from the Arabs. In them were concealed matters coming from the wise men of our age, and this splendid knowledge of the expert was not even looked at by the eye of the untutored. Now when I saw such splendid wisdom placed in front of (restored to) you in an ugly setting ... I cleansed it from the hand of the Gentile, and wrote it out in the Holy Language, which is so dignified in tone.[19]

Thus, he composed the following works: 1. *Mishlei Shuʿalim* (Fox Fables), a collection of 119 fables, largely drawn on the Aesopic fables in their different medieval versions. A similar version in old French or Anglo-Norman was produced by Marie de France who was active as a poet in the second half of the 12th century. The earlier assumption[20] that Berakhyah was inspired by this French version is, according to Golb, unlikely.[21] Berakhyah's special endeavour with his *Fox Fables* was, as Golb puts it, "to produce a Hebrew Ysopet of elevated taste, with which he wanted to make accessible in Hebrew a product of non-Jewish culture that he believed could have value for the Jews of his milieu."[22] In order to "Judaise"[23] the material at hand, to purify it from its ugly, i.e. pagan elements, Berakhyah eliminated all mythological and pagan references, as well as the deities mentioned in his prototypes. 2. Two

---

[19] Trans. and ed. H. Gollancz, *Dodi ve-Nechdi* (Uncle & Nephew), Oxford 1920, p. 16.

[20] Cf. Hadas, *Fables of a Jewish Aesop*, pp. v–ix; A.M. Habermann, *Mishlei Shuʿalim le-Rabbi Berekhyah ha-Naqdan*, Tel Aviv-Jerusalem 1945–1946, pp. v–viii.

[21] Cf. Golb, *The Jews in Medieval Normandy*, p. 339.

[22] Golb, *The Jews in Medieval Normandy*, pp. 340–341.

[23] Term derived from Haim Schwarzbaum, *The Mishle Shuʿalim (Fox Fables) of Rabbi Berakhyah ha-Nakdan. A Study in Comparative Folklore and Fable Lore*. Kiron 1979, p. xxv.

religious-ethical treatises, one entitled *Sefer ha-Mazref*, and a second treatise which the editor Gollancz called "Ḥibbur" (Compendium) as he could not find a title for it,[24] but which probably carried the name *Musar* or *Musar Haskel ("The Discipline of Wisdom")*, following the reconstruction of the title from the colophon of the Vatican manuscript by Golb.[25] Both works are largely an adaptation and summary of religious ideas expressed by Saʿadya Gaʾon in his *K. al-Amānāt wa l-Iʿtiqādāt* (Book of Beliefs and Opinions), which was accessible to Berakhyah in the old, unprinted Hebrew paraphrase. Other secondary sources consulted by him are Baḥya ibn Pakuda and Solomon ibn Gabirol. In this way Berakhyah transmitted basic ideas of Muslim *Kalām* philosophy as above all expressed in Saʿadya's *Book of Beliefs and Opinions* to a Jewish public. 3. *Sefer Dodi we-Nekhdi* or *Sheʾelot* mentioned above, a Hebrew adaptation and paraphrase of the *Quaestiones Naturales*, a popular twelfth century book on the natural sciences composed by Adelard of Bath which belongs to a genre called "Masāʾil wa-ajwiba" in the Arab literary tradition, and especially reminds one of the so-called "Problemata physica", which study the reasons and causes of phenomena in nature.[26] 4. *Sefer Koʾaḥ ha-Avanim*, see below. Finally, Berakhyah also played a prominent role in promoting knowledge of the Jewish tradition by commenting on the books of the Bible, especially by explaining difficult terms and translating them into Old French.[27]

3. Sefer Koʾaḥ ha-Avanim (On the Virtue of the Stones)

This work composed by Berakhyah at an unknown date is extant in a single manuscript, namely Oxford Bodleian Library, Can. Or. 70, cat. Neubauer 1147, fols. 73a–80b, which was copied in an Ashkenazi script in the fourteenth century.[28] The text featuring in the margin of a liturgical

[24] Cf. Gollancz, *The Ethical Treatises of Berachya*.

[25] Golb, *History and Cultute of the Jews of Rouen*, p. 137; idem, *The Jews in Medieval Normandy*, p. 345.

[26] Cf. H. Daiber, entry "Masāʾil wa-adjwiba" *Encyclopaedia of Islam*, new ed., vol. 6, pp. 636a–639b.

[27] Cf. Golb, *History and Cultute of the Jews of Rouen*, p. 124ff.; idem, *The Jews in Medieval Normandy*, pp. 333–338.

[28] Cf. Ad. Neubauer, *Catalogue of the Hebrew Manuscripts in the Bodleian Library*, Oxford, Clarendon Press, 1886, repr. 1994. And: *Supplement of Addenda and Corrigenda* compiled under the direction of Malachi Beit-Arié and edited by R.A. May, Oxford: Clarendon Press, 1994.

text has been copied by a scribe who hardly new any Hebrew and did not understand the text at all, so that it is replete with mistakes and corruptions. Recently, the text has been published anonymously in an anthology of 29 Hebrew texts on precious stones entitled: *Sefer Segullot ha-avanim ha-ṭovot.*[29] Unfortunately, this edition is uncritical and replete with mistakes. Berakhyah's lapidary, allegedly the oldest Hebrew lapidary that has come down to us,[30] received much attention in the past because it contains possibly one of the earliest references to the sailor's compass in the following passage describing the stone called "aimant" (magnet stone):

> There is one variety of it (i.e.magnet stone) which the seamen carry with them, because owing to it they know, when they drift on the sea, which way leads in the right direction, for it attracts the iron. They put a needle in the water and the stone next to it, and the needle rushes to the stone by virtue of its force. But the diamant, because of its superior force, takes the needle away from it.[31]

The book describes 72 stones which are arranged in alphabetical order as is common for lapidaries, with the exception of stones 68 to 70. The virtues of the stones are of a medical-scientific character and/or of a magical-supernatural one; we do not find any reference to allegorical or astrological connotations of the stones. These virtues can be activated in essentially two different ways, either by external application of the stone to the body just like an amulet, or by internal application in case the stone is friable. In the case of external application the stone can be worn by putting it in a bag and hanging it around the neck or by setting it in a ring or necklace. If the stone has a hole it can be attached with a thread to the body. Thus, Berakhyah remarks in the case of the onyx (5) that it "induces dreams in everyone who wears it on his finger, but if he hangs it around his neck he is visited in his dreams", and the crystal (57) is said to be beneficial for a woman suffering from a difficult childbirth if attached to her leg, suspended by a woolen thread. Next to these common methods of external application one also finds other ones, as in the case of the magnet stone (1) of which it is said that "Magicians carry it with

---

[29] Ed. Jerusalem 2005.

[30] Cf. Steinschneider, *Lapidarien*, p. 62.

[31] Cf. I. Löw, *Mineralien der Juden*, p. 132, in: *Fauna und Mineralien der Juden*. Herausgegeben und mit einem Vorwort und Anmerkungen versehen von A. Scheiber, Hildesheim 1969; Steinschneider, *Die hebräischen Übersetzungen im Mittelalter und die Juden als Dolmetscher*, p. 964, remarks that the text only refers to the magnet needle and not to the compass.

them to be used in their deeds. The one who carries it with him will not dream when he is asleep. It protects from all reptiles, calms wrath and appeases quarrels. It makes wise the fools, and keeps the enemies away. Its force [is active] when one carries it in his hand or in the left wing(?) of his garment." When the stone is applied internally, its powder is imbibed with a liquid like a medicinal powder, alternatively one may rinse the stone with a liquid and then drink it. For instance, for redness of the eye it is recommended to leave a beryl (28) in water for one night and then to rinse one's eyes with that water.

Such detailed descriptions and stipulations of the actual application of precious stones go back to Dioscurides, *Materia Medica*, which was composed between 50–70 CE and not only describes the medicinal properties of plants but also those of around two hundred stones in book five.[32] Following Dioscurides these different ways of application became part and parcel of ancient and medieval lapidaries in general.[33] Thus, they feature in the description of minerals and gemstones by Pliny the Elder (23–79), whose *Natural History*, Books 36 and 37 drawing on a wide variety of sources became one of the most influential sources for medieval stone lore. Next to the applications mentioned above, Pliny describes some novel ones, such as stones that are not ingested as a powder, but to be carried in the mouth, and stones to be attached to the body with the hair of a certain animal.[34] These traditions recur in later lapidaries, including that by Berakhyah who relates about the "alectorie" (alectorius) (no. 3):

> Whoever carries it defeats his enemies in war, wherefore ancient kings used to wear it. Possessing it increases wealth, and merchants who carry it are successful and return home. Whoever wears it will not be thirsty, and who carries it between his teeth will please everyone. It arouses sexual desire, fills ⟨...⟩ (the brain: trans. Marbode), and is beneficial for a woman in hard labour. Ladies wear it to please men, and it is extremely powerful when one carries it in his mouth.

Likewise it is stated of the gelacia (44) which looks like hail and is always cold that if you put it in your mouth at midday at the time of the New

[32] Cf. M. Wellmann, Pedanii Dioscuridis Anazarbei. De Materia Medica. Libri quinque. Repr. Berlin 1958; J. Berendes, *Des Pedanios Dioskurides aus Anazarbos Arzneimittellehre in fünf Büchern*. Übersetzt und mit Erklärungen versehen, Stuttgart 1902, repr. Wiesbaden 1970.

[33] Cf. Joan Evans, *Magical Jewels of the Midle Ages and the Renaissance particularly in England*, Oxford 1922. Repr. London 1976, p. 16; Paul Studer and Joan Evans, *Anglo-Norman Lapidaries*. Paris 1924. Repr. Genève 1976, p. x.

[34] Evans, *Magical Jewels of the Midle Ages and the Renaissance particularly in England*, p. 17.

Moon, you will know future events. And the tradition to attach the stone to the body by means of a hair features in the description of the chrysolite (29): "The one who wears it need not fear wild animals. If you find it pierced, pass a hair from the tail of an ass through the hole: it is then beneficial for madmen, to bring them back to their mind," and also in that of the chalcedon (58).

Most the stones described in Berakhyah's lapidary are effective through their intrinsic power which can be activated by men through their mere external or internal application. However, in the following tradition related in the lapidary (29) the power can only be activated through certain magical formulas which should, perhaps as stones are difficult to write on, be written on the object in which one carries it: "If someone who goes to the council wears it (i.e. the chrysolite) around his neck [inserted] in the skin of an unborn deer he will not die. He should write on it [i.e. on the skin]: Oshie[l], Baʿadie[l], Havhie[l] provide me with assistance." And in the case of the unidentified stone called "Periṭora" (52) it is stated that the formula ṬiBaQoṬ QWṬNY should be written on the silver ring in which the stone is set, as these names are tried [as beneficial] for gout, also when one does not use the stone.

According to some historians such an object should not be called amulet, but talisman, as it has letters or words inscribed on it.[35] And in a tradition about the topas (40) the magical practice of interiorising the power of the stone by drinking wine with which the stone has been rinsed is associated with that of inscribing magical formulas on a piece of parchment and drinking it: "One should wash it in wine three times a day, in the evening, morning and afternoon, and drink [the wine]. One should [also] write on parchment: ʾNQ, YWD(?), ṬRYP, PṬYR, ʾWGʿ, then wipe out what is written in wine, and drink this". These kinds of magical practices which intended to transmit the charm in physical form were, as Trachtenberg remarks, common practice in medieval love charms.[36] In the Jewish tradition examples of this practice are found especially in the context of recipes for forgetfulness, as in Ḥayyim Vital's "Practical Kabbalah and Alchemy":

[35] Cf. R. Kieckhefer, *Magic in the Middle Ages*. Cambridge, p. 77; G. Bos, "Jewish Traditions on Strengthening Memory and Leone Modena's Evaluation", *Jewish Studies Quarterly*, vol. 2,1,1995: 39–58, p. 42.

[36] J. Trachtenberg, *Jewish Magic and Superstition. A Study in Folk Religion*. 1939. Repr. New York 1975, p. 123.

> Take three leaves of the Rubus sanctus (ṣeneh), on the first leaf write TTYTYTYH; on the second SSS, and on the third leaf PPPYH; erase the names with wine or water and drink this. Even if one has only learned *Ḥumash*, his heart will be opened (the common expression used for the ability to remember) so that the miracle will be great.[37]

These magical practices in which certain formulas or letters had to be written on stones in order to activate their power originated in Alexandria in the second century where many treatises recording these practices are based upon *litteromancy*, and are divided into twenty-four chapters, each corresponding with a letter of the alphabet. The most important treatise of that kind is the so-called Kyranides, of which the prologue states the first book to be the work of Cyranus King of Persia. It became influential through the Latin translation by Gerard of Cremona in 1175.[38]

It should be noted that in some cases Berakhyah's lapidary not only describes the way in which the stone is to be applied but also stipulates physical and psychical conditions, as in the description of the agate (2), where it is said that "Everyone who wears it with a whole heart and with true understanding will be comforted of his grief," while of the beryl (28) and jasper (41) it is stated that its wearer has to be pure. In the case of some stones, such as the emerald (4), chalcedon (58) and calcofanus (60) it is stipulated that one should not have sexual intercourse while carrying them. Such stipilations feature in other texts on precious stones as well. Thus, the 13th century exegete, preacher and kabbalist Baḥya ben Asher ben Ḥlava states in his Torah commentary in the section on the twelve precious stones which were part of the breastpiece of the high priest: "I saw in the *Book of Stones* composed by the philosopher [i.e. Aristotle] that stones require purity. Well-known is their special property that if someone wears a stone while he is impure their power is abolished or weakened. But if he repents and becomes pure, the stone regains its former power." The same quotation with a kabbalistic argumentation features in an anonymous text entitled "Avnei ha-ḥoshen lefi shemot ha-shevaṭim" (The stones of the breastpiece according to the names of the twelve tribes) which is extant in MS Paris BN hebr. 1284, fols. 145a–146a.[39]

---

[37] Cf. G. Bos, Ḥayyim Vital's "Practical Kabbalah and Alchemy": a 17th Century Book of Secrets, p. 60; for earlier traditions see idem, Jewish Traditions on Strengthening Memory and Leone Modena's Evaluation, pp. 42–43.

[38] Evans, *Magical Jewels*, pp. 17–19; Studer-Evans, *Anglo-Norman lapidaries*, p. xi.

[39] Quoted following the anonymous collection of texts on precious stones, ed. Jerusalem 2005, p. 101.

If we look at Berakhyah's lapidary from a statistical, medical point of view, it is clear that stones beneficial for women's diseases feature most frequently, namely ten times, followed by those for eye diseases (eight times), bleedings (seven times), poisons and poisonous reptiles (six times), epilepsy (five times), gout and swellings (four times).

4. *The Source(s) of* Sefer Ko'aḥ ha-Avanim (On the Virtue of the Stones)

When looking into the source(s) of Berakhyah's lapidary the first thing to take into consideration is that of the nature of this particular literary genre in general which has been characterised by John Riddle in the following words:

> One is immediately struck by the remarkable variations among the lapidaries in the information concerning what is presumably one stone. In fact, hardly any two lapidaries among the many hundreds are alike. Far from relying entirely on classical authorities, the lapidarists often felt obligated to relate their own experiences about the wonderful effect of stones. When one becomes aware of the large number of stones and variations, sometimes contradictions, in information about them, it is obvious that the compiler exercised personal judgment of some kind in determining what to put into his particular text.[40]

To make his point Riddle gives us a concrete example of the various traditions of the emerald as they exist in the medieval lapidary literature.[41] The texts belonging to this genre are not static but variable, fluid, changeing all the time, as the compiler(s) would add or delete as they saw fit. And this holds good also for the copyist(s) as we shall see in the case of the anonymous *Ellu shemot ha-avanim ha-ṭovim*, that is the Hebrew prose translation of Marbode of Rennes' *De lapidibus*.[42] The eclectic character of lapidaries may also explain why research sofar has only given us general and vague indications of the possible sources of this lapidary.

[40] J. Riddle, "Lithotherapy in the Middle Ages. Lapidaries Considered as Medical Texts," in: *Quid pro quo: Studies in the history of drugs*, Hampshire 1992, p. 50.

[41] Riddle, *Lithotherapy in the Middle Ages*, pp. 47–50.

[42] Ed. John Riddle, *Marbode of Rennes' (1035–1123) De lapidibus. Considered as a medical treatise with text, commentary and C.W. King's translation, together with text and translation of Marbode's minor works on stones* (Sudhoffs Archiv. Beihefte, Heft 20). Wiesbaden 1977. Recently, a new edition has been published by Maria Esthera Herrera, *Lapidario. Liber lapidum*, Paris 2005.

Thus, Renan-Neubauer remark that it is a translation of a French or Latin lapidary;[43] Gross remarks that he does not know its sources as there existed many lapidaries in Berakhyah's time.[44] Steinschneider surmises that the original should be looked for in Romance literature.[45] Gollancz suggests that he translated from a French source from which he copied verbatim the French words as in the text before him.[46] Habermann states that it is a translation-adaption of a Latin book about the magical powers in stones.[47] In his monograph on the Jews of Rouen Golb remarks that Berakhyah's lapidary is neither identical with that composed by Marbode of Rennes, nor similar to it in its contents,[48] and in his more recent monumental monograph on the Jews in medieval Normandy he states that according to Steinschneider this lapidarium was translated literally from a Latin or French work, but that a prototype of this kind has never been discovered.[49] However, the anonymous editor(s) of the collection of Hebrew lapidaries intimated a close relationship between Berakhyah's lapidary and that composed by Marbode, as they stated that *Ellu shemot ha-avanim ha-ṭovim* drew amongst others drew on Berakhyah's lapidary.[50] Our research into the possible sources of Berakhyah's lapidary has indeed confirmed a connection between the two texts insofar as both have Marbode as a common source. Marbode (ca. 1035–1123) was born in Angers, France, where he became master of the cathedral school c. 1067 and chancellor of the diocese of Angers c. 1069. In 1096 he became archbishop of Rennes in Britanny. His *De lapidibus* written in Latin hexameters and drawing on a wide variety of sources, such as Damigeron, Dioscurides, Pliny, Isidore of Seville, Solinus, and Costa ben Luca,[51] was the most popular medieval book on stones surviving in not less than 160 manuscripts.[52] It was, moreover,

---

43 E. Renan-A. Neubauer, *Les Rabbins français du commencement du quatorzième siècle*. Paris 1877. Repr. Farnborough 1969, p. 496.

44 Gross, *Gallia Judaica*, p. 180.

45 Steinschneider, *Lapidarien*, p. 62.

46 Gollancz, *The ethical treatises of Berakhyah*, p. XXIX.

47 Habermann, *Berakhyah Ben Natronai ha-Nakdan*, col. 596.

48 Golb, *History and Cultute of the Jews of Rouen*, p. 134, n. 373.

49 Golb, *The Jews in Medieval Normandy*, p. 343.

50 Ed. Jerusalem, p. 7.

51 See Riddle, *Marbode of Rennes*, pp. 8–21.

52 Herrera, Lapidario, pp. xviii, ci–cxvi. In his edition of the Latin Marbode Riddle (p. ix) refers to 125 manuscripts amongst a total of 616 medieval lapidary manuscripts, while in "Lithotherapy in the Middle Ages" (p. 44) he remarks that he found 137 manuscripts of *De lapidibus* alone.

translated into virtually all European languages, such as French, Provençal, Italian, Irish, Danish, Hebrew, Spanish, Castilian, and Dutch.[53]

Especially the French translations and adaptations of Marbode are of prime importance since both the Hebrew translations, that is the anonymous *Ellu shemot ha-avanim ha-ṭovim* and the verse translation prepared by Jacob Ben Reuben, and Berakhyah consulted these versions, and not the Latin ones. These medieval French versions were composed in Anglo-Norman England, the earliest, the socalled First French Version of Marbode's Lapidary before 1150, to be followed by three more versions which are called the "Second and Third Prose Lapidaries" and the "Second Lapidary of Engraved Gems". Soon after their composition they spread beyond the island into continental France.[54] The version which Berakhyah consulted more than any other for the composition of his stonebook is the Cambridge Version of Marbode which was made directly from the Latin text and is not dependent, like the other Anglo-Norman versions, on the First French Version.[55] The Cambridge Version was Berakhyah's main source for at least 43 of the 72 stones featuring in his lapidary, as is shown in the supplement in the detailed analysis by Julia Zwink.

As to the Hebrew translations, the anonymous translation starting with: *Ellu shemot ha-avanim ha-ṭovim koḥam we-ẓeva mar'ehem u-gevuratam be-tavnitam* (*These are the names of the precious stones, their virtues, colors, powers and shape*) is extant in MS Bern, Burgerbibliothek 200.2 which was copied in an Ashkenazy semi-cursive script in the year 1290. The text features on fols. 104a–108b, while the text featuring on fols. 109b–111b contains a discussion of some engraved stones, partly agreeing with Arnaldus Saxo "De gemmarum virtutibus".[56] This manuscript is characterized by numerous short additions in both margins and in the text itself, as noted above. A second copy of this translation can be found in MS Oxford, Bodleian Heb. d. 11 (cat. Neubauer-Cowley 2797/45),[57] fols. 352a–358b. It was copied by Eleazar ben Asher ha-Levi

[53] Cf. Evans, *Magical Jewels*, p. 34; Studer-Evans, *Anglo-Norman lapidaries*, p. xv.

[54] Studer-Evans, *Anglo-Norman lapidaries*, pp. xix–xx.

[55] Cf. Studer & Evans, *Anglo-Norman lapidaries*, p. 154.

[56] See Olivia Franz-Klauser. *Burgerbibliothek Bern. Die hebräischen Handschriften. Verzeichnis mit Einleitung*. Zürich 1999. For the text from Arnoldus Saxo, cf. E. Stange (ed.), *Die Encyklopädie des Arnoldus Saxo, zum ersten Mal nach einem Erfurter Codex herausgegeben* (Königliches Gymnasium zu Erfurt. Beilagen), Erfurt 1905–1907, pp. 75–77.

[57] A. Neubauer and A.E. Cowley, *Catalogue of the Hebrew Manuscripts in the Bodleian Library*. Vol. 2, Oxford 1906.

in an Ashkenazy script in the fourteenth century,[58] and ends, contrary to the previous manuscript, with the following excipit: סליק ספר האבנים הנקרא בלשון לטין לפדריוש (This is the end of the stonebook which is called "Lapidarius" in Latin). This manuscript was used for the uncritical and faulty edition in *Sefer Segullot ha-avanim ha-ṭovot* mentioned above. An indication for the fact that this text is not derivative upon a Latin Marbode Vorlage but a French one are some Old French terms which it shares with French versions of Marbode's Lapidary. Two examples are: namely לו⟨ב⟩א צֵרְבא or לוטא צרבא (MS Oxford) for luve cervire,[59] i.e. lynx, and לֵימַצון or לימצון (MS Oxford) for limaçun, i.e. tortoise.[60] Since the anonymous translation is just like Berakhyah's lapidary derivative upon the old French versions of Marbode's lapidary its readings closely parallel those by Berakhyah in the case of several stones.[61] In some cases this translation has been used to emend corruptions and to clarify obscure terms or passages in Berakhyah's text.

The Hebrew verse translation by Jacob ben Reuben entitled "Sefer ha-'Osher" is extant in the following manuscripts: 1. Bibliotheek der Rijksuniversiteit te Leiden Cod. Or. 4763 (Warn 25),[62] fols. 115a–119b; 2. Rome, Biblioteca Casanatense 3082/11, fols. 107a–115b; 3. St. Petersburg, Russian National Library Evr. I 677, eighteenth century; 4. London, British Library Or. 10721; 5. New York, Jewish Theological Seminary, Ms. 2542; 6. New York, Jewish Theological Seminary, Ms. 2733.[63] The text has been edited in *Sefer Segullot ha-avanim ha-ṭovot* on the basis of the Leiden manuscript, but suffers from mistakes. According to Steinschneider Jacob ben Reuben is not identical with the author of *Sefer Milḥamot ha-Shem* (The Book of the Wars of the Lord), the anti-Christian polemic composed in 1170.[64] However, Judah Rosenthal, the editor of the book, tends to affirm the identity.[65]

---

58 According to Eli Yassif, *Sefer ha-zikhronot*, Tel Aviv 2001, the scribe is possibly the son of one of the copyists of the Bern manuscript. I thank Binyamin Richler for this note.

59 Cambridge Lapidary, ed. Studer-Evans, p. 176, l. 600.

60 First Prose Lapidary, ed. Studer-Evans, p. 106, no. 29.

61 For an impression of the similarity between the anonymous translation and Berakhyah's lapidary see the comparative table in the supplement.

62 M. Steinschneider. *Catalogus Codicum Hebraeorum Bibliothecae Academiae Lugduno-Batavae*. Leiden 1858.

63 For these data cf. the online catalogue of Microfilmed Hebrew Manuscripts at the Jewish National and University Library.

64 Steinschneider, *Die hebräischen Übersetzungen im Mittelalter und die Juden als Dolmetscher*, p. 957.

65 Rosenthal, *Ya'aqov Ben Re'uven. Sefer Milḥamot ha-Shem*. Jerusalem 1963, pp. x–xi.

5. *The Critical Edition of* Sefer Ko'aḥ ha-Avanim

The critical edition is based on the Hebrew text as it features in the margin of the Oxford manuscript. As the text contains many corrupt and hard to read passages and words, it has been emended throughout, when possible on the basis of secondary material, amongst which ancient and medieval lapidaries such as Pliny, Damigeron, Arnoldus Saxo, Marbode's Latin text and French translations and the anonymous Hebrew prose translation with which Berakhyah's text shares several terms and even passages, as we showed in the comparative table following in supplement 2. The question of the relationship between Berakhyah and the anonymous Hebrew Marbode prose translation lies beyond the scope of this edition and might never be answered unequivocally, as we do not know the identity of the author of the translation, nor the date of composition.

6. *Supplements*

The first supplement consists of a comparison between the text of some stones as it features in Berakhyah's stonebook and that of the anonymous translator of the stonebook by Marbode of Rennes.

The second supplement prepared by Julia Zwink consists of the following items:

1. A general introduction to the Old French terms, written in Hebrew characters, in Berakhyah's lapidary.
2. A linguistic study of the graphical / phonological and lexicological aspects of every single Romance / Latin term.
3. Berakhyah's sources.
4. Tables of the sources.
5. Glossaries.
6. Bibliography and abbreviations.
7. Subject index of English and foreign terms.

TEXT AND TRANSLATION

These are the virtues of the stones,
compiled by R. Berakhyah, of blessed memory

1 **Aimant**[1] is their name, and their hues fall into four classes. They are found in mines of gold, silver and copper. The hard variety is called *diamant*,[2] and I will treat it with God's help.

The *magnetes*,[3] which belongs to this variety, is known to attract iron. There is one variety of it which the seamen carry with them, because owing to it they know, when they drift on the sea, which way leads in the right direction. They put a needle in the water and the stone next to it, and the needle rushes to the stone (North)[4] by virtue of its force.[5] But the *diamant*, because of its superior force, takes the needle away from it.

Magicians[6] carry it with them to be used in their deeds. The one who carries it with him will not dream when he is asleep. It protects from all reptiles, calms wrath and appeases quarrels. It makes wise the fools, and keeps the enemies away. Its force [is active] when one carries it in his hand or in the left wing (sleeve?) of his garment.

2 **Acates**:[7] it is so called after a river from which it is won, and which is in the land of *Sezile*.[8] It is black as a raven and has a white circle around it, encircled by a brim. Embedded in it are various kinds of shapes, which are not man-made. Kings of old used to wear it, because it is very powerful in battle and also because their seal was made of it, [showing that] no hands interfered with it to engrave it.

In the land of *Crete*[9] the *coral*[10] stone is found, which resembles it [lit. them], except that it has hues similar to gold. It is very precious and is called the treasure [*segullah*] of kings. He who wears it need not fear nor serpent, nor scorpion, nor any reptile. Some have forms like that of boughs from woods, some have the form of desert creatures. Some satiate

---

1 *Aimant* is O. Fr. for 'diamond' and 'magnetite'; also cf. Riddle, *Marbode*, no. 1 and entry no. 38. For references and linguistic analyses for all the O. Fr. terms within the Hebrew text, see Supplement B-2.

2 *Diamant* is O. Fr. for 'diamond'.

3 *Magnetes* is Lat. for 'magnetite'.

4 Gad Freudenthal suggests to read the Hebrew האבן as הצפ⟨ו⟩ן, i.e. 'the North'.

5 Cf. Introduction to this volume.

אילו כח האבנים מיסוד הר׳ ברכיה נקדן מנוחתו כבוד

1 אַאִימַנְט שמם ומראי⟨הם⟩ נחלקים על ארבע עינינים. והם ימצאו במקורת זהב וכסף ונחושת. המין הקשה שבה נק׳ דְיַאמַנְט ובו אדבר בעזר ד׳.

ואבן מַגְנֵיטְיש, שהיא מן מינה, ידועה שמושכת הברזל. ויש בו מין אשר חובלי הים ישאוה כי בעבורה ידעו איזה הדרך יש בו הרוח בתעותם בים [כי היא מושכ⟨ת⟩ הברזל]. והם נותנים מחט במים והאבן אצלה, והמחט רצה אל האבן בכחה. והנה הדְיַאמַנְט [כי] בכחו העודף עליה יגזול ממנה המחט.

וחוברי חבר ישאוהו להעזר בפעולתם. ואשר ישאנה עליו, בשכב⟨ו⟩ לא יחלום חלום. ומצלת מכל זוחלי עפר, משככת חמה, ומריבה משקטת. ומחכמת המשוגעים, מרחקת האויבים. וכחה לשאת א⟨ו⟩תה ביד או בכנף חלוקו השמאלי.

2 אקטץ. הנהר אשר יוציאו זה ממנו נקרא בו, והוא בארץ שְזִילְא . שחור הוא כעורב וסביבה עוגל לבן אשר זר לו סבי⟨ב⟩. וכמה מיני צורו⟨ת⟩ נמצאים בה בלא מעשה ידי אדם. ומלכים קדמונים הורגלו לנשאה כי כח גדול יש לה במלחמה, וגם כי חותמם ממנה ולא חלו בה ידים לפתח פתוחה.

ובארץ קְרֵיטְא נמצא אבן קוֹרָל הדומה להם, אך כי יש בה גוונים דומים לזהב. והוא יקר מאד, וקראוהו סגולת מלכים. הנושאו לא יירא מנחש ועקרב, ולא מכל זוחלי עפר. יש בהם מצורות ענפי יער, ויש בה⟨ם⟩ צורתם חיות מדבריות, יש מהם משיבים

---

2 בעזר: emendation editor בעזך MS   5 האבן: = הצפ⟨ו⟩ן?   11 לו: emendation editor לא MS   12 חותמם: emendation editor חותמה MS   14 אבן: emendation editor אבל MS   15 מנחש: emendation editor מנפש   16 חיות (= A) emendation editor את MS

---

6 Cf. Deut. 18:11.

7 *Acates* is O. Fr. for 'agate'; also cf. Riddle, *Marbode*, no. 2: "a variety of chalcedony with patterns of bands, irregular and variegated in appearance, which can produce images of faces, woods, animals, etc."

8 *Sezile* is the O. Fr. name for 'Sicily'.

9 *Crete* is the island 'Crete' in O. Fr.

10 *Coral* is O. Fr. for 'coral'.

the soul longing for water, some afford light to dim eyes. Some of them emanate an odor that is as good as spices burning in the fire. The one who wears it pleases those who see him. Everyone who wears it with a whole heart and with true understanding will be comforted of his grief.

3 ***Alectuene** (*alectoire*):[11] Three years after the castration of the cock this stone, which is named after it, grows close to its stomach. No species of stone is comparable to it if it is removed from the cock at the right time, which is seven years after the castration, [at which time] it is full-grown. The largest one resembles a bean which is called *feve.*[12] Its aspect is white, like crystal, but not through and through. In some cocks it is found in the intestines, in others around the hip, in others in ⟨…⟩.

Whoever carries it defeats his enemies in war, wherefore ancient kings used to wear it. Possessing it increases wealth, and merchants who carry it are successful and return home. Whoever wears it will not be thirsty, and who carries it between his teeth will please everyone. It arouses sexual desire, fills the brain, and is beneficial for a woman in hard labour. Ladies wear it to please men, and it is extremely powerful when one carries it in his mouth.

4 **Esmeralde:**[13] This stone exists in twelve varieties of color. Some can be found in copper mines, namely those in which there are stains, like bright spots on the skin. The best amongst them is that which, when you look at it, is completely green, without any whiteness in it. This green is dark [thick?] as leek—which is called **porels (porreus)*[14]—, but [the stones?] are pure and shiny according to their dimness [opaqueness] and lustre [?]. The choicest ones come from the land of **Ciie (Cithie).*[15]

The inhabitants of the island called "Gryphons" go and surround an island whose inhabitants is a nation called "Arismapi", who have neither a head nor a brain, but have one eye on the chest. Those called "Gryphons" wait in ambush for the people called "Arismapi" when they collect the stones from the profound depths [of the sea], and [rob] them of their stones.

---

[11] *Alectoire* is O. Fr. for 'alectorius'; for the identity of this stone, cf. Riddle, *Marbode*, no. 3: "Doubtlessly the "stone" was a bit of gravel found in the gizzards of cocks."

[12] *Feve* is O. Fr. for 'bean'.

[13] *Esmeralde* is O. Fr. for 'emerald'. The original term "smaragdus" could be any green

נפש שוקקה למים, יש מהם מאירות עינים כהות, יש מריחות מהם ריח טוב כבושם בוער באש. הנושאה ימצא חן בעיני רואיו. ויתנחם מצערו כל נושאה בלב שלם ובדעת נכונה.

3 אַלֵיקְטוּיְנָא. אחר שלש שנים לסירוס התרנגול זאת האבן ששמה בו צומחת קרוב לקורקבן. וכל המינים לא ישוו בה אם נלקחת מן התרנגול בעתה, שזהו אחר שבע שנים אחר סירוסו, היא | נגמרת כולה. הגדולה כעין מיני קיטנית שקורי⟨ם⟩ פיבא. ותארה לבן כעין קרישטל אך לא מכל וכל. ויש תרנגול שנמצאת במעיו, ויש סביב הירך, ויש על .... fol. 73b

הנושאה ינצח אויביו במלחמה, ועל כן מלכים קדמונים נשאוה. מחזקת העושר בחזקתו, והסחרים מצליחים ושבים לביתם בנשא אותה. המשימה לא ⟨י⟩צמא, והנשאה בין שיניו ימצא חן בעיני כל. מעירה התאוה, ממלאה המוח, וטובה למקשה לילד. והגבירות ישאוה למצא חן בעיני האנשים, ועוצם גבורתה לנשאה בפיו.

4 אֶשמרַלדְא . זאת האבן אשר תמצא על שנים עשר מיני⟨ם⟩ במראה.

יש אשר תמצא במקורו⟨ת⟩ נחושת, והם א⟨ו⟩תם אשר תמצא בם כתמים כמו בהרות. והטובה מהם היא כשתרא⟨ה⟩ אותה ירוקה מכל וכל, בלא לובן בתוכה. והירוק עב כמו כרתי שקורי⟨ם⟩ פורלש, אבל זכות ומאירות לפי עבי ויהרה [= זהרה?]. ומארץ שאיאה (= שיטאה?) באות המובחרו⟨ת⟩.

ויושבי האי הנקרא גריפונש הולכים וסבבים אל אי אחת אשר יושביה אומה אחת הנקרא ארישמפי, ואין להם לא ראש ולא מוח, אך עין יש להם על החזה. ואותם הנקרא גריפונש יארובו על האומים הנקרא ארישמפי בלקטם את האבנים במצולות עמקי תהום ⟨...⟩ האבנים מהם.

---

1 מריחות: emendation editor מריקות MS   4 לקורקבן: emendation editor לקורקבו MS
5 שקורי⟨ם⟩: emendation editor שיקורי MS   11 גבורתה: emendation editor גערתה MS גבורתו
A 15 שקורי⟨ם⟩: emendation editor שיקורי MS   18 מוח (= A): emendation editor מום MS

---

stone in the Middle Ages and in antiquity, such as green marble, alabaster, serpentine or aquamarine; cf. Riddle, *Marbode* no. 7.

14 *Porreus* is O. Fr. for 'leek'.

15 *Cithie* is Angl.-Nor. for Scythia.

Since this stone is good, the[16] sun does not warm it, and it shines even in the dark. If you find in it a concavity, you can see your face in it, just as you see your reflected image in the water. But the perfect [stone], without cavity, is better than it, and the eye takes pleasure in looking at it. A king called "Nero" had such a stone, a very large one, at which he used to look when his army was fighting and he would [fore]see the victory.

[If] one keeps it in purity, without getting defiled in intercourse with women, [then, as long as he carries it with him, ⟨…⟩[17] sexual lust. Through [this] stone one's wealth[18] increases and does not diminish. He who wears it around his neck will speak well, and will respond to everyone as he sees fit. In times of thunder it has the capacity to take away fear. It is also good for meetings because it pleases. Someone suffering from a hot disease [fever] or from epilepsy should wear it around his neck. He who wants to preserve the color of this stone, should [wash] it in wine and then rub it with verdant olive oil.

5 **Onicle:**[19] This stone induces dreams in everyone who wears it on his finger, but if he hangs it around his neck he is visited in his dreams. It arouses anger, insolence and strife toward anyone who carries it. If one hangs it around the neck of a child, it will spit out saliva and phlegm. [But] without doubt, if one sews it into the skin of a miscarried lamb and hangs it around the neck of the child with a single thread, that child will not cry without reason, and will not fear the evil eye and a sudden terror.[20]

This stone can be found in five varieties. If one such stone is found that overcomes [lit. bends] another stone which is called *sardine*,[21] then it is the very best; it takes then away the fear and evil brought about by fear that we have mentioned.

The [stone] that hails from India is red as blood, and has a white brim all around. And the [variety] that comes from Arabia is black and has a white brim. This [stone] is beneficial for cavities in the teeth to alleviate the pain. [It is also beneficial] to undo the witches' [evil] eye from the bewitched: if it is rubbed with goat's milk, and the milk is drunk, the spell is undone.

---

16 "the sun does not warm it, and it shines even in the dark": cf. A: "If this stone is [exposed to] the sun, the latter neither covers its appearance nor darkens its colors (i.e. it still glitters and shines)."

17 "⟨…⟩ sexual lust": "overcomes the lust for fornication" A.

18 "wealth": "glory" A.

והנה האבן הזאת, בהיות⟨ה⟩ טובה, השמש לא יחם, וגם בחשך מאירה. ואם תמצא בה מקום אחת שקוע תוכל לראות פניך בו כאשר תראה צילך במים. אך השלמה בלא חלל טובה הימינה, והעין תתענג במבטה בה. מלך הנקרא נירוש היה לו כזאת האבן גדולה מאד אשר בה היה מביט בהלחם צבאו ורואה הנצחון.

⟨...⟩ שומר זאת בנקיות בלי להתגאל במשכב הנשים, כל זמן שהוא נושאה עליו, ⟨...⟩ תאות המשגל. ובה יעדיף הונו ולא יפח⟨ת⟩. ונושאה בצוארו יכול לכלכל דבריו במשפט לענות כל איש ואיש כחפצו. טובה בעת הרעם להסיר הפחד, וטובה לוועד כי היא נושאת חן. ומי שיש לו חולי חם או נכפה ישאנה בצוארו. והרוצה לשמור מראה זאת האבן ⟨ירחצנה⟩ ביין ואחר ימשחנה בשמן זית ירוק.

fol. 74a 5 אוניקלא. זאת האבן תעורר החלומות לכל אשר נושאה באצבעו, | אבל אם יתלה אותה בצוארו אז יפקד בחלומו. מעוררת כעס ועזות פנים ומריבה לכל נושאה. והתולה אותה בצואר הילד יוציא ריר וליחה מפיו. ובלא ספק התופרה בעור טלה נֵפֶל, ויתליה בו בחוט אחד בצואר הילד, אותה הילד לא יבכה בחינם ולא ירא מעין רע ומפחד פתאום.

וזאת האבן תמצא על חמשת מינים. ואם ימצא באבן הזאת שהיא מכפפת [מ]אבן אחרת הנקר⟨את⟩ שַרְדִינְא אז היא טובה מכל וכל. ואז תסיר הפחד וכל רוע הפחד שדברנו.

הבאה מארץ אנד⟨י⟩ה אדומה הי⟨א⟩ כדם וזר לבן ⟨לה⟩ סביב. והבאה מארץ הערב שחור וזר לבן לה. ואותה טובה לחפור השינים להסיר הכאב; ולהסיר מבט מכשפות מן המכושפים אם ימחו אותה בחלב עיזים וישתו ויתיר הכשוף.

---

1 בהיות⟨ה⟩ טובה, השמש לא יחם וגם בחשך מאירה: בהיות אצל השמש לא יחפי ראותה ולא יאפיל מראיה A 6 ⟨...⟩ תאות המשגל: ומנצחת תאות הזנות A‖ הונו: הודו A 7 לוועד emendation (A =) לייעד MS editor 9 ⟨ירחצנה⟩: = A 10 אוניקלא: emendation editor אזניקלא MS 18 וזר: emendation editor וזה MS

---

[19] *Onicle* is O. Fr. for 'onyx'; also cf. Riddle, *Marbode*, no. 9.
[20] Cf. Proverbs 3:25: אל תירא מפחד פתאום (You will not fear a sudden terror).
[21] *Sardine* is O. Fr. for 'sard'.

6 Etite:[22] There are two varieties [of this stone]. The red ones are called "male" and the white ones "female". This is a precious stone.

It can be found in the great sea that is called *occian*[23] or in the kingdom of Persia, in eagles' nests. For the eagle carries it into the nest of its fledglings because the power of this stone protects them so that they do not go outside the nest and fall to the ground.

The term "etite" means 'pregnant' in the language of that country. For [this stone] contains within it another stone and if you shake it you can hear from the outside the sound of the stone in it like [that of] a bell. This stone is doubtlessly powerful, for in a house in which it is a woman will not miscarry. Therefore the women of Salerno wear it while they are pregnant.

The one who carries it on his left side will defeat his enemies and increase his wealth. It heals epileptics. If someone doubts whether or not a person hates him and he fears that that person might poison his beverage or food, and he wants to test whether this person hates him, he should invite him to eat with him from the same bowl of good food and place this stone in the bowl without that person's knowledge. Then, if that person hates him and intends to harm him he will not be able to eat anything from that food. But once he removes the stone, he will eat immediately.

There were twins in the land of Arabia who wore that stone by their father's order so as to remain healthy.

7 Heliotrope:[24] This is a good and precious stone. Its lustre tends somewhat towards the green of the emerald stone. If someone puts it in a water vessel, it changes the sunlight so that it becomes red like blood. If you put it in a vessel full of water, the water will boil as if by fire. It changes the fair weather so that it may rain. When it is outside of water, it captures the sunlight [so that] you notice it during a solar eclipse. The one who wears it knows future things and can foretell them.

---

[22] *Etite* is O. Fr. for 'aetits, eagle-stone'; the identity of this stone is uncertain; T.G.H. Drake, "The eagle stone, an antique obstetrical amulet"; *Bulletin of the History of Medicine*, 8 (1940): 128–130, p. 128, referring to T.J. Pettigrew, *On superstitions connected with the history and practice of medicine*, London, 1844, remarks that it is "a composition of the oxyde of iron with small portions of silex and alumina, which rattle within upon being shook …"; according to D. Wyckoff, Albertus Magnus. *Book of Minerals*. Oxford 1967, it is "a hollow geode or concretion containing loose cristals, pebbles, or earth". Riddle,

6 אִיטִיטְא. שני מינים יש בהם. האדומו⟨ת⟩ נקרא⟨ות⟩ זכרים והלבנות נקבות. זאת ⟨אבן⟩ יקרה.

ובתוך ים הגדול הנקר⟨א⟩ אוֹקְצִיַּאן או במלכות פרס תמצא [או] בקן הנשר, לבעבור כי הנשר ישאנה בקן גוזליה לבעבור כי כח זאת האבן שומרת אותם פן יצאו חוץ לגבול הקן ולא יפלו על הארץ.

ולשון אטיטא בלשון הארץ ההיא הרה, לפי שאבן אחרת יש בתוכה וכשתנענע א⟨ו⟩תה בחוץ תשמע קול האבן אשר בתוכה כפעמון. כח האבן הזאת רב בלי ספק כי האשה לא תפיל בבית אשר היא שם. על כן ישאוה עליהן נשי שלירנא כשהן הרות.

הנושאה בצד שמאל ינצח אויביו ומרבה הונו ומרפאה הנכפי⟨ם⟩. ומי שיש לו ספק על איש אם ישנאהו אם לא ומתיירא ממנו פן ישקנו או יאכילנו סם המות וירצה לבחנו אם שונא הוא לו יזמיננו לאכול עמו בקערה אחת ממאכל טוב וישי⟨ם⟩ זאת האבן בתוכה בלא ידיעת האי⟨ש⟩. אם שונאו וחושב להרע לו לא יוכל לטעום מאומה מן המאכל ההוא, ובע⟨ת⟩ יסיר האבן יאכל מיד.

ושני תאומים נמצאו בארץ הערב נושאי א⟨ו⟩תה האבן במצות אביהם כדי לשמרן בבריאות.

7 אאליוטרופא. זאת האבן טובה ויקרה. ונוטה קצת זוהרה לירוק של אבן אישמרלדא. מי שמשים א⟨ו⟩תה בכלי מלא מים מחלפת אור השמש ומתחלף אורו כאודם דם. ואם תשימנה בכלי מלא מים אז יעל⟨ה⟩ רתיחות כמפני האש. ותשנה האויר בעת שקט להמטיר. וכשהיא חוץ מן המים מקבלה אור השמש ותבחין | בה בעת קדרות השמש. fol. 74b
מי שנושאה עליו ידע מן העתידים וידבר עליהם.

8 כן: emendation editor כל MS   18 בכלי: מים scribal addition and deletion   19 השמש: תשמיש scribal error השמש scribal correction

Marbode, no. 25, states that "there is today a brown, iron mineral stone in a seventeenth century silver mounting with the word aetites inscribed on it in an 18th c. hand," and that "the inscription adds that it is to be held in childbirth".

[23] *Occian* is Angl.-Nor. for 'ocean'.

[24] *Heliotrope* is O. Fr. for 'heliotrope'. This is our bloodstone, a dark chalcedony with red spots of jasper; cf. Riddle, *Marbode*, no. 29.

He who wears it on one of his fingers will attract glory and honor and health on himself as long as he wears it. It stops bleeding: when one puts some of the blood on the stone and dries it in the sun or on a fire it stops the bleeding. There is a homonymous herb [such that] the one who knows [the appropriate] incantation over both of them can take as he pleases wealth from its owner and he will not say a thing.

[These stones] can be found in the land of Africa, Ethiopia and Cyprus.

8 **Abeste:**[25] It is unique, no stone is like it. In the land of Arcadia you will find its color to be like blood. It is very pure. It cools iron and all kinds of hot metals—when they glow it stills them. It has the power to protect all tree-fruit from worms, and avoid that they suffer damage from water. If you look at it against the sun, it emits such a strong red glow that the eye cannot contain it. Its power [comes to bear] when held in the left hand.

9 ***Ematice (ematite):**[26] The Arabs (= Greeks?) named it thus in their language because it somewhat resembles rust of iron.[27] It has the power to alleviate disease and pain. It heals eye illness: when one touches one's eyelids with it, and having his eyes red like mutton, he should take some of its powder together with egg white, mix them well and put it on the eyes, and he will be healed. If you look [at it] against the sun, you see sparks in it, red like blood. This is why the Arabs named it in their language after the name of dragon-blood (?). Physicians who have some of this stone make from it a **collyriu* (*collyrium*).[28]

Someone who spits blood should finely grind the stone and touch it [= the powder]. If someone immerses it in water, that water will heal dry and wet eczema. If someone hides it in his hair or puts it under [...], he will understand a spell pronounced over him, be it good or bad. If a woman suffering from [excessive] menstruation drinks the water, her flux will stop. For dead flesh in the living being it is beneficial to strew on it the powder. To stop diarrhea, one should dilute the stone in old wine and drink it. One who has been bitten by a serpent or any reptile should

[25] *Abeste* is O. Fr. for 'asbestos', (from Gr. ἄσβεστος, 'incombustible'): According to Riddle, *Marbode*, no. 33, the term refers to "a group of different minerals with similar appearances," and "the best known source of asbestos is a form of serpentine known as chrysolite."

ומי שנושאה באצבעו ימשוך הוד וכבוד עליו ובריאות כל ימי היותה עליו. ומעמדת זוב הדם; בתת מן הדם על האבן וייבשנו לשמש או לאש אז יעמד לדם. ויש עשב ששמו כשמה, להיודע ללחוש על שניהם יוכל לקחת הון כחפצו לפני בעליו ולא ידבר מאומה ובארץ ארפיק וכוש וציפרא ימצאו.

8 אֲבִישְׁטא. יחידת היא, שאין אבן דומה לה. ובארץ ארקדיו תמצא מראה שלה כעין דם. והיא זכה מאד. ברזל וכל מיני מתכות חמ⟨ות⟩ תקרר בזריחתם תשקיטם. כחה לשמור כל פרי העץ מבלי תתליע, גם לא יזיקנו מים. או שיביט בה נגד השמש יצא זוהר ממנה כאש אדום מאד עד אשר לא תוכל עין לשלוט בו. וכחה ⟨...⟩ לשאת א⟨ו⟩תה ביד שמאל.

9 אֵימַטִיש. קראוה כן ההגרים (= הגרקים?) בלשונם לפי שקצת דומה לחלד ברזל. כח יש לה להקל חלי ומדו⟨ה⟩. ולחולי עינים תרפא: מי שיגיע זאת האבן בעפעפיו— ולפי שעיניו אדומות כבשר שׁוֹר—יקח מן האבק עם חלבון ביצה ותערב יחד היטב וישים על עיניו וירפא. וכשתביט בה נגד השמש תראה בה ניצוצות אדומות כדם, על כן קראוה הערביים על שם דם תנין בלשונ⟨ם⟩. והרופאים שיש להם קצת ⟨מ⟩האבן יעשו ממנה קולירִיו.

ומי שמוציא דם מפיו יכת הדק מן האבן ויגע בה. ומי שישרנה במי⟨ם⟩, אותה המים ירפאו גרב יבש ולח. הטומנה תחת שערו או נותנה תחת ⟨...⟩ יבין מה שלוחשין עליו, אם לטובה אם לרעה. והאשה זבה אבל תשתה המים תעצור זיבותה. ולבשר המת שבחי טוב האבק לזרוק עליו. ולעצור שילשול ימסוך האבן ביין ישן וישתהו. ומי שנעקץ מנחש

1 ימשוך: emendation editor ימשיך MS 5 ארקדיו: emendation editor אוקורט? MS 8 תוכל: emendation editor תכלה MS 9 שמאל: emendation editor שאול אל MS 14 קצת: emendation editor קאת MS 18 תעצור: emendation editor תעש MS

[26] O. Fr. *ematite* (from Gr. αἱματίτης for 'bloodstone'), is our hematite, a red oxide of iron; also cf. Riddle, *Marbode*, no. 32.

[27] Cf. Marbode, ed. Riddle, l. 467: Sumpsit emathites Grecum de sanguine nomen (The Hoematite—named by the Greeks from blood—).

[28] *Collyrium* is Lat. for 'eye-salve' (Gr. κολλύριον).

wash the wound with the water [in which the stone was diluted] and he will be cured. And someone who has [...] with water [...].[29] This stone is found in Ethiopia, Arabia and Africa, this is where it is mined.

10 **Abeste:**[30] Its luminousness is like that of of pure (unadulterated) iron. This stone is found in Arabia,[31] and is highly marvelous. He who kindles it, will dispose of an eternal flame that he will not be able to extinguish. He who has this stone does not need even a single candle.

11 ***Exacratlitu (exacontalithos):**[32] [This is] a very precious stone, in which there are sixty colors, but which is extremely small. Although small [in size], it is yet very large in vigor, for all the powers found in the other stones are present in this stone. The people called "Tragtodes" (= Troglodites) bring [these stones with them] from the land of the Lybians.

12 **Orite:**[33] This is a round black stone that is very good. Its power is to heal wounds inflicted by wild animals. If someone pulverizes it with rose water and drinks it, it will heal his wounds. He who carries it, need not fear [wild] animals.

There is a second variety of this stone, whose lustrousness tends towards green and which has stripes around it. He who carries it will not suffer downfall.

There is yet a another variety of this stone whose lustrousness tends towards green and which has stripes around it, but it is very bad. For a woman who wears it will be barren; and if she had worn it before conceiving [and then got pregnant] then she will have a miscarriage.[34] [This stone] is smooth on one side, and rough on the other. Therefore, warn every woman against wearing it.

---

[29] Cf. A: "He who suffers from stones in the bladder should drink it with water, and the stones will dissolve in the water."

[30] Cf. entry 8.

[31] "Arabia": "Arcadia" Marbode, ed. Riddle.

או מכל זוחלי עפר ירחץ הפצע מהמים וירפא. ומי שיש⟨...⟩ במים ⟨...⟩. ובארץ כוש וערב ואפריק תמצא זאת האבן ומשם תוצאותיה.

10 אֲבֵיִשְׁט. זוהרה כברזל נקי. וזאת האבן בארץ הערב, ונפלאת היא מאד. כי מי שידליק אותה אש תמיד תוקד [לו] אשר לא יוכל לכבות. ומי שיש לו האבן—נר אחד לא צריך.

fol. 75a **11** אֵיקְשַׁקְרַטְלִיטו. אבן יקרה מאד ויש בה ששים גוונים | אבל קטנה היא מאד. ואם היא קטנה, גדולה היא מאד בגבורתה, כי כל כחו⟨ת⟩ שימצאו בשאר אבנים ימצאו בזאת האבן. והאומים הנק׳ טְרַגְטוֹדֵיש יביא⟨ו⟩ם מארץ הלובים.

12 אוֹרֵיטא היא אבן שחורה ועגולה וטובה מאד. גבורת⟨ה⟩

לרפאות פצעים שנפצעו מחיות יער . מי שיכתתנה עם מי שושני⟨ם⟩ וישתה המים, ירפא את פצעיו. ומי שנושאה עליו לא ייִרא מחי⟨ו⟩ת.

ויש עוד מין שיני מזאת האבן, נוטה זהרה לצד ירוק וסביב לה חברברות. לא יפול מי שנושא זאת האבן עליו.

ועוד ימצא בה מ⟨י⟩ן אחר מזאת האבן, נוטה זהרה לצד ירוק וסביב לה חברברות, אבל היא רעה מאד. כי אשה הנושאה עליה לא תוכל ללדת, ואם היא נ⟨ו⟩שאה בטרם תתעבר תפיל מן הוולד. מצד אחד היא חלקה ומצד השיני מלאה שערו⟨ת⟩. ולכך הזהר כל אשה מלנשא⟨ה⟩.

---

1 ירחץ הפצע (= A) editor emendation ירפא MS ‖ ומי שיש⟨...⟩ במים ⟨...⟩: ומי שיש לו אבן במקוות השתן ישתה האבן במים וימס האבן במים A   2 זאת: editor emendation פאת? MS   3 זוהרה: editor emendation זיהרה MS ‖ הערב: ארבנדימא A m Arcadia   4 שידליק אותה editor emendation שידליקנה A שיקליד אותה MS   10 יער: editor emendation תער MS רעות A

---

[32] M. Lat. *exacontalithos* (from Gr. ἑξηκοντάλιθος for 'sixty stones in one' because of its many colors) is probably our opal, cf. Riddle, Marbode, no. 38 (following Eichholz, Pliny, Natural History XXXVII, 60, 167).

[33] *Orite* is O. Fr. for 'oritis'. The identification of this stone is uncertain; cf. Riddle, *Marbode*, no. 43.

[34] The text may be corrupted and perhaps should read: For if a woman wears it she will not be able to conceive, and [if a pregnant woman] wears it before she has given birth, she will have a miscarriage.

13 Enidre:[35] In the eyes of all scholars this is a wondrous stone, for it continually weeps and [exudes] tears in any circumstance.[36] It is unknown why, given that it is very hard. No one knows its nature. For just as abundant water gushes out of a spring [without exhausting it], so also water gushes out of it, [and yet] its thickness does not diminish and all the water that flows out of it does not empty it.

14 *Ematice (ametiste):[37] Its essential luminousness is like that of the flower of peaches, called *pesques*[38] in a foreign language, or like that of the flower of violets. It was called so [i.e. **ematice*] because its color to some extent tends to [that of] blood, for ἆιμα is blood in the language of the Greeks.[39]

There is one variety that resembles the stone called **zonce (jagonce) grenat*,[40] [and another] variety in which there are [figures of?] roses. And there is a variety that is somewhat whitish, like red wine mixed with water. There are [altogether] five varieties [of this stone].

It is soft and easy to quarry. Its main power is that someone who wears it will not get drunk. It elicits favor and is useful to [...] for skillful hunters, fieldmen,[41] for they will be successful in their hunting. Its appearance somewhat resembles that of the stone called *sarde*.[42]

15 Alemandine:[43] This stone hails from the land Almedine.[44] Many err with respect to its appearance. Most of them are hollow in their lower part, and burn like coal. We do not know all of its virtues, but he who wears it will not fear a deadly poison or a harmful potion. If you put it in cold water, it will warm up.

---

[35] *Enidre* is O. Fr. for 'enhygros' (⟨Greek ἔνυδρος for '[stone] with water inside'), which is possibly chalcedony containing water; cf. Riddle, *Marbode*, no. 46.

[36] Cf. Isaiah 25: 8.

[37] *Ametiste* is O. Fr. for 'amethyst'; also cf. Riddle, *Marbode*, no. 16.

[38] *Pesques* are 'peaches' in O. Fr.

[39] ἆιμα is Gr. for 'blood'. The etymology given by Berakhyah is not that of the amethist, but of the hemathite, cf. entry 9. The correct etymology of amethist is from Greek ἀμέθυστος, meaning 'not drunk'.

[40] *Jagonce grenat* is O. Fr. for 'garnet red jacinth'.

[41] Cf. Gen. 25: 27.

13 אֲנִידְרָא. זאת האבן נפלאת בעיני כל החכמים, יען כי היא בוכה לעולם ודמעות על כל פנים. ולא נודע למה, לבעבו⟨ר⟩ כי קשה היא מאד. ולא ידע איש תולדתה, כי כאשר יצאו מים רבים ממקור המעיין יצאו ממנ⟨ה⟩ מים, לא תפחת מן עביה ולא תורק מכל המים שיצאו ממנה.

14 אֵימַטִישְׁא. עיקר זהרה כפרח אפרסקין, פֵּישְׁקְשׁ בלע⟨ז⟩, או כפרח עשב וִיאלַטְא. ולפי שקצת מראיתה נוטה לדם קראוה כן, כי אֱמַה הוא דם בלש⟨ון⟩ הגר⟨ק⟩ים.

ויש מ⟨י⟩ן אחד הדומה לאבן הנקר⟨את⟩ צונצא (?) גרנט, או מין אשר בו שושנים. ויש מ⟨י⟩ן אחד קצת לבנה כיין אדו⟨ם⟩ שנתערב בו מים. ובהם נמצאו חמשה מינים.

והיא רכה וקלה לחצוב. עיקר גבורתה שלא ישתכר הנושאה. ונושאת חן, וטובה לעשות [...] אל יודעי ציד אנשי שדה כי יצליחו בצידתם. תארה ⟨דומה⟩ קצת לאבן הנק׳ שֵׂרְדְא.

15 אַלְמְדִינְא. זאת האבן באה מארץ אלמדי⟨נא⟩ והרבה ישגו במראיתה. ורובם חלולות בתחתיהם ודולקות כגחלים. לא ידענו כל גבורתה, אך הנושאה לא יירא מסם המות וממשקה לרע. ואם תשימנה במים קרים יחמו.

3 רבים emendation editor יבין MS   5 זהרה: emendation editor זהרת MS   6 אֱמַה: emendation editor אֱמֵד MS   11 הנק׳: emendation editor בנקר׳ MS   12 והרבה: emendation editor להרבה MS

[42] *Sarde* is O. Fr. for 'sard, a variety of reddish calcedony'; also cf. the description of next stone.

[43] *Alemandine* is O. Fr. for 'alanbandica, alemandine'. Originally a variety of carbuncle (cf. Pliny, *Natural History* 37.25.96) this term changes later to give us our almandine, which, according to Wyckoff, *Albertus Magnus*, p. 72, "mineralogists apply to a garnet, and jewelers also to a spinel, of a very dark purple-red color"; see as well Riddle, *Marbode*, no. 21.

[44] Cf. Marbode, ed. Riddle, ll. 330–331: Est Asiae regio, quae nomen habens Alabanda fert alabandinam, cuius lux emula Sardi (From Asia's climes rich Alabanda sends the Alabandine; In fiery lustre with the Sard it vies).

16 Yenia:[45] We do not know where [this stone] comes from. Many say that it is found in the eyes of an animal called *hyaena*.[46] For from the eye of this animal they take the pupil, which is in the center of the whole eye. In a few days it becomes as hard as other stones. It is very pure. He who wears this stone can foretell the future as he wishes, if he washes this stone and puts it under his tongue. Therefore, the ancient generations said that it makes one into a prophet.

17 *Irone (iris):[47] This stone hails from the Red Sea. Its color is like that of the crystal. The Arabs love [this stone] and fetch it from the sea. It always has six sides (hexagonal). If one holds it up in a house against the rising sun, [i.e. with the sun] shining opposite to him, he will see on the walls of the house a few colors, like those of the rainbow in the sky. Its virtue is to give [victory] in war, and on account of its great virtue it has been called **irone*.[48]

18 *Andro dragaza (*androdragma*):[49] You find it in the sand on the seashore. Its appearance is like that of refined silver. It is as hard as the diamond. It is good to calm wrath and anger.

19 *Optallies (*optallie*):[50] This stone has the power to heal the eye with the water in which it has been washed. Thieves wear it while they search houses, for it affords them light in the dark and they see all that is in the house. But those who are in the house do not see or notice them. The [thieves] thus take whatever they wish.

20 Absite:[51] It is black with red [veins]. It weighs more than anything[52] of the same size. If someone heats it in fire a single time, it remains hot for seven whole days.

---

[45] *Yenia* is Lat. for 'hyaena-stone'. This stone is hard to identify. Wyckoff, *Albertus Magnus*, p. 96 remarks that it perhaps an "eye agata", chalcedony with concentric rings of different colors; however, following Pliny's description (*Natural History* 37.60.168) she remarks that it is more likely to be an iridescent or chatoxant mineral. Riddle, *Marbode*, no. 44, suggests that it is rather an agate with patterns resembling an eye.

[46] *Hyaena* is Lat. for 'hyaena'.

[47] O. Fr. *iris*, 'iris', is derived from Greek for 'rainbow': according to Riddle, *Marbode*, no. 47, it is "a transparent quartz crystal."

[48] This term is difficult to identify; cf. the discussion in Supplement B-2.

16 אֵינִיאָה. לא ידענו מאין תב⟨ו⟩א. ורבים א⟨ו⟩מרים כי נמצאת בעיני חייה ששמה איניאה, כי מעין החיה יקחו ב⟨ב⟩ת | עין, הממוצעת בתוך כל העין. ובימים מועטים fol. 75b
תהיה קשה כשאר אבנ⟨ים⟩. והיא זכה מאד. הנושא זאת האבן יוכל לבו ⟨לדעת⟩ העתידות כחפצו, ברחוץ זאת האבן וישימנה תחת לשונו. ע״כ אמרו דורות הראשונ⟨ים⟩ שהיא עושה אדם נביא.

17 אִירוֹנָא. זאת האבן באה מים סוף וכאבן קרישטל מראה. והערביים א⟨ו⟩הבין אותה ומביאין אותה מן הים. ולעולם נמצאו בה ששה קצוות. מי שיאחז בה בבית נגד זריחת השמ⟨ש⟩ מנֻגַהַ נגדו יכול לראות בקירות הבית כמה גוונים, כמראה הקשת אשר בשמים. כחה לתת ⟨ניצחון⟩ במלחמה, ובעבור גודל כוחה קראוה אירונא.

18 אַנדְּרוֹ דְרַגְצָא. בחול של שפת ים תמצא מראיתה ככסף מזוקק וקשה כאבני אאימנט וטובה לשכך אף וחימה.

19 אופטליאש. זאת האבן כחה לרפ⟨אות⟩ העין במי רחיצתה. והגנבים בעת יחתרו בתים ישאוה, לפי שהיא תאיר להם בחשך ויראו כל אשר בבית, ואותם שבבית לא יראום ולא ירגישו בם, ויקחו כל חפצם.

20 אַבשִׁיטְא. שחורה היא, וגוונים אדומות יש בה. והיא שוקלת יותר מכל דבר שגדול כמוה. מי שיחם אותה באש פעם אחת תהיה חמה כל שבעת הימים.

1 ששמה: emendation editor שמומה MS 3 תהיה: emendation editor תהיון? MS 6 אותה emendation editor אותם MS 7 אותה: emendation editor אותם MS ‖ ששה: emendation editor עשה MS ‖ שיאחז בה: emendation editor שיאברו? MS שיאחזנה A 9 כוחה: emendation editor אותה MS 12 יחתרו: emendation editor יסתברו MS 15 מכל דבר: emendation editor הכל דברי MS מכל דבר שגדול כמוה: מדבר גדול ממנה A

---

[49] Lat. *androdragma*, (variant of *androdmas*, from Gr. ἀνδροδάμας, 'man-tamer'); cf. Pliny, *Natural History* 37.54.144. s.v. androdamas. It is probably our pyrite, see Riddle, *Marbode*, no. 48.

[50] *Optallie* is O. Fr. for 'opal'; also cf. entry no. 22.

[51] *Absite* is O. Fr. for 'apsyctos', which is possibly lignite or anthracite coal, and as a hard gem anthracite; cf. Riddle, *Marbode*, no. 42.

[52] "anything of the same size": "anything that is larger than it" A.

21 Electrum:[53] It looks like wax. If one sets it alight, it burns like a torch. Its opaqueness [i.e. transparence] is the same as that of [rock-]crystal, and it attracts straw.

22 *Uptalus (*optallius*):[54] This stone has dissimilar colors. Its name is like that of a city in the land of India. Some of it are luminous like a flame, and thereby resemble the carbuncle, while the vigor of its luminousness is similar to that of the aematite. It also has a green [tint] like the emerald.

He who wears it will be cured from eye-ache. If he is a thief, he will not be caught while he still wears it. And if he is imprisoned in iron chains, he will be able to free himself.

23 *Ancotre:[55] It somewhat resembles [rock-]crystal but it is not as transparent. Its size is that of a small nut. A woman who wears it will not miscarry. If someone wants to test its virtue, he should hang it around the neck of a hen. Etc.

24 *Asistos:[56] It is a green [stone]. The one who wears it, need not fear sorcery.

25 *Ansra (*ambra*):[57] It hails from the intestines of a large sea fish called *baleine*.[58] It is transparent, pure and yellowish, its luminousness somewhat resembles liquid honey. If you ignite it, it burns like a candle. It is useful to wear it in order to be safe from evil spirits.

When fumigated, it stops [excessive] menstrual flow of a woman, [namely] when the smoke [coming] from it penetrates her [i.e. the womb], and the woman who suffers from intestinal pain should drink from the water in which it [had been immersed] for a day or a night. Its fumigation is good for headache.

If you chew between your teeth the [kind] that is intermediate between white and black, it will stick to your tongue and fill the mouth with good odor. This is the choicest.

---

[53] *Electrum* is Lat. for 'amber'; cf. *Albertus Magnus*, ed. Wyckoff, p. 121; Marbode, ed. Riddle, no. 59, discusses the criselectrus (golden-electrum).

[54] *Optallius* is Lat. for 'opal'; also cf. entry 19.

[55] This stone could not be identified with certainty. The Hebrew term is perhaps a corrupt transcription of Lat. *acintitota*, 'hyacinthe'.

[56] This stone could not be identified; it is perhaps Lat. *apsyctus*, (from Gr. ἄψυκτος for 'uncooled stone)' (cf. entry no. 20).

21 אֱלִיקְטְרוּם. כשעוה תארה. ואם נתן עליה אש בערת כלפיד. ועבה היא ⟨כ⟩קרישטל, ומושכ⟨ת⟩ אליה הקש.

22 אֻופטלוּש. זאת האבן גוונים משונים לה, ושמה כשם עיר אשר בארץ אינדא. יש בה במקצתה זוהר שלהב⟨ת⟩ אש, ומזה דומה לקַרְבּוּנְקַל, ועוצם זהרה דומה לאבן אימטיט. ויש בה ירוק כעין אַשְׁמַרַלְדָא.

מרפא הנושאה מכאב העינים. ואם הוא גנב לא יתפש בעודה עליו, ואם נאסר בכבלי ברזל יוכל להסירם מעליו.

23 אַנְקוּטְרא. דומה קצת לקרישטל אך אינה צלולה כל כך, ומדתה כאגוז קטן. אשה הנושאה אינה מפלת. והרוצה לנסות כחה יתלנה בצואר תרנגולת, וג׳.

24 אַסְצְטוּשׂ. ירוקה. הנושאה לא יירא כישוף.

25 אַנְסְרַא. באה ממע⟨י⟩ דג גדול שבים הנקר⟨א⟩ בַּלֵינָא. והיא | צלולה וזכה וצהובה, fol. 76a
קצת דומה זהרה לנופת דבש. ואם תשים בה אש דולקת כנר. טובה לשאתה להנצל מרוח רעה.

והיא בעישונה תעצר זיבות האשה כאשר בא העשן מתוכה לתוכה, והאשה שנכאבו דקיה תשתה מן המים אשר ⟨הושמה⟩ בתוכה יום אחד או לילה. והעישון טוב לכאב הראש.

ואותו שהוא ממוצע בין לבן לשחור, אם תלעסנו בין שניך ודבק בלשונך ומלאה הפה מריח טוב, והוא המובחר.

1 אֱלִיקְטְרוּם: emendation editor אֱלִיקְטְרוּמ MS 12 לנופת: emendation editor לשפת MS
14 בא: emendation editor באה MS

[57] Lat. *ambra* is missing in Marbode. Although not a stone in our text, the term *ambra* probably also means, just like the Arabic parallel *'anbar*, 'amberstone'; cf. Ruska, J., *Das Steinbuch des Aristoteles. Mit literargeschichtlichen Untersuchungen nach der arabischen Handschrift der Bibliothèque Nationale* herausgegeben und übersetzt. Heidelberg 1912, pp. 56–57, 154, no. 14; G. Bos and G. Mensching, "Shem Tov Ben Isaac, Glossary of Botanical Terms, nrs 1–18", *Jewish Quarterly Review*, vol. XCII, July–October 2001: 1–20, pp. 26–27.

[58] *Baleine* is O. Fr. for 'whale'.

When the lust of women to sleep with men becomes very strong and they cannot [do] as they desire, they put it deep in that place [i.e. the vagina] in order to cool the heat of their lust, for it has the power to discharge from them the [female] seed.

26 Asterites:[59] Light is enclosed in it, seemingly moving within it like the light of a star. It turns the sun's brilliance into white.

27 *Amauntes (*amiantus* (?)):[60] Its [color] is intermediate between black and red. It relieves the body. If you mix its powder with egg white, it alleviates the illness of the eyelids and enlightens the eyes [i.e. improves eyesight].

It is very good to drink for someone who ingested a deadly poison. It pulverizes the stone in the urinary bladder.

28 Beril:[61] It is somewhat white, and that whiteness is greenish; its color is close to that of sea water. [Stone] cutters make it with six facets. It has the power to draw a man's love to his wife. If someone wears it when he is pure, his eminence will increase.

[If held] tightly in the hand one can get burnt and scorch his palm, because the warmth of the flesh activates it until it becomes hot.

To cure the redness of the eye, one should leave it in water for one night and rinse his eyes with that water. If someone daily drinks water in which it was immersed it will free him from sighing and cure him from pain in the liver. With that water one can restore one's eyesight as it was when he was young. He who suffers from gout should touch the affected spot [with this stone] and he will be cured. If you hold this stone against the sun, you can ignite a piece of cloth or ⟨...⟩. Many said that he who wears it will not drown.

29 Grisolite:[62] Its color is like that of the sea, and within it there is what looks like a gold granule: it turns and twists here and there according to how the eye looks at it. When it is set in pure gold, its hue is like that of a burning coal. When it is in the shade you can distinguish in it a green color.

---

59 *Asterites* is Lat. for 'chatoyant'; it does not feature in Marbode, but for a close parallel cf. Supplement B-3.

60 This stone could not be identified; the Hebrew term is similar to Lat. *amiantus* (Pliny

נשים כשתגבר תאותן לשכיבת האנשים ולא יוכלו ⟨לעשות⟩ כחפצן, משימות אותו בעומק המקום ההוא, לקרר חום תאותן, כי בו כח להפליט הזרע מהן.

26 אֵישְׁטְרִיטַשׁ. אור מוסגר בה, ו⟨מ⟩תהלך בה כאור הכוכב לפי מרא⟨ית⟩ העין. והופכת זריחת השמש ללובן.

27 אַמַאְוּנְטְשׁ. ממוצעת בין שחו⟨ר⟩ לאדום, מנחמת הגוף. וכאשר תער⟨ב⟩ עפרה עם לובן ביצה תקל חולי עפעפים ומאירה העינים.

טוב מאד לשתות למי שאכל סם המות. והיא תפוצץ האבן אשר במקוה השתן.

28 בֵּירֵיל. קצת לבנה, ואותו הלובן יתייחש קצת לירוק, וקרוב מראהו למי הים. והחוצבין עושין בה ששה קצוות. כחה להמשיך אהבת הבעל אל אשתו. והנושאה בנקיות יגדל כבוד⟨ו⟩.

⟨והמחזיקה⟩ בידו בחזק יוכל ליכוות בה ולשרוף כפו, לבעבור כי חום הבשר יעוררינה, עד שתחם לו.

ולהסיר אודם העין יניחנה במים לילה אחת וירחץ עיניו מן המים. והשותה מי שריתה בכל יום יסיר אנחות לבו וירפאינו מכאב הכבד. ומן המים ההם ישיב אור עיניו כימי עלומיו. ומי שיש לו גוטָא יגע במקום החול⟨י⟩ וירפא. כשתשים זאת האבן נגד השמש [עד] תוכל להבעי⟨ר⟩ האש בבגד או ⟨...⟩. ואמרו רבים כי לא יטבע הנ⟨ו⟩שאה.

29 גְרִיזוֹלֵיט. עינה כעין הים ובתוכ⟨ה⟩ כגרעין זהב, סובב לפי מראה העין בה ופונה אנה ואנה. וכשהיא משבצת בזהב מזקק ⟨עינה⟩ כגחל בוער. וכאשר ⟨היא⟩ בצל תוכל לראות בה עין ירוק.

2 תאותן: emendation editor מאותן MS 7 במקוה: emendation editor במקלת MS 13 שריתה: emendation editor שהיתה MS 14 עיניו emendation editor פניו MS 16 הנ⟨ו⟩שאה: emendation editor הנשאר MS

XXXVII, 31, 139)/ *amiantos* (Isidore, *Etymologies* XVI, 4, 11), 'a kind of asbestos'. However, this stone has different properties.

[61] *Beril* is O. Fr. for 'beryl'; cf. Riddle, *Marbode*, no. 12.

[62] *Grisolite* is O. Fr. for 'chrysolite' (from the Gr. χρυσόλιθος meaning 'golden stone'); it is the stone which is now called olivine by the mineralogists and peridot or chrysolite by the jewellers; cf. Riddle, *Marbode*, no. 11.

The one who wears it need not fear wild[63] animals. If you find it pierced, pass a hair from the tail of an ass through the hole: it is then beneficial for madmen, to bring them back to their mind. One who was stabbed with a sword should hold it in his hand: if he vomits, he will die; if not, he will live. If a man whose fortune turned from good into bad wears it, he will regain his good fortune and he will be successful as long as he wears it. It is beneficial to look at it in the morning.

If someone who goes to the council wears it around his neck [inserted] in the skin of an unborn deer he will not die. He should write on it [i.e. on the skin]: Oshie[l], Baʿadie[l], Havhie[l], provide me with assistance.

He who suffers from nightmares should wear it [encased] in a ring of tin or lead on his left hand.

30 **Grisoprase:**[64]: Its color is like that of leek soup, with sparks of gold glistering in it. It is beneficial for an epileptic: as long as he wears it, he will not fall. It is beneficial for [someone suffering from] **ortice (artetice)*[65] to wash this stone in water and drink the water.

31 ***Grisopacion (crisopacion):**[66] In the dark you can perceive its luminousness, but during the day you do not discern luminousness in it. It alleviates thirst and comforts the mind.

32 **Gagatromé:**[67] By its spots it resembles the hair [pelt] of a lamb. The one who wears it will be dreaded by his enemies. An ancient king used to wear it in battle, and was victorious as long as he wore it; one day he forgot [to wear] it and was killed.

33 **Galactites:**[68] It is somewhat green, and the green is of a somewhat dark shade. And if you look closely—its color is like ashes of trees.

A woman who wants to have much milk should pulverize this stone in whey[69] and drink this [potion] immediately after bathing, before she eats anything else: it tastes like milk, and also looks like it. If someone weaves a thread from the wool of an ewe, perforates this stone, and hangs it around her neck with this thread, she will have plenty of milk. If she [the ewe]

---

63 "wild animals": A reads: "evil spirits".

64 *Grisoprase* is O. Fr. for 'chrysoprase' (from the Gr. χρυσόπρασος meaning 'golden leek green') it is a variety of chalcedony, cf. Riddle, *Marbode*, no. 15; also cf. entry no. 31.

65 *(Gute) artetice* is O. Fr. for 'gout'.

66 *Crisopacion* is M. Lat. for 'chrysoprase'; see previous stone no. 30.

הנושאה לא יירא מחיה רעה. ואם תמצאנה נקובה שים בנקובת שיער מזנב חמור, אז טובה למשוגעים להשיבם אל דעתם. מי שנדקר בחרב יקחנה בידו, ואם יקיא ימות ואם לאו יחיה. | fol. 76b והאיש אשר נהפך מזלו מטוב לרע, אם ישאנה ישוב לקדמתו, ויצליח כל זמן שהיא עליו. וטובה להביט עליה בבקר.

ומי שהולך לבית הוועד, אם ישאנה בצווארו בעור צבי הנמצא בבטן אמו לא ימות. ויכתוב בו: אושיא בעדיא הבהיא היו לי למסעד.

ולאשר חלומות יבעתוהו ישאנה בטבעת בדיל או עופרת ביד שמאל.

30 גְרִיזוֹפְּרְש. כמרק כרת מראה, אך כעין ניצוצי זהב ינוצצו בה. טובה לנכפה, לא יפול בעודה עליו. וטובה לאוירטץ לרחוץ זאת האבן במים וישתה המים.

31 גרישופציאון. בחשך תוכל להכיר זהרה, אך ביו⟨ם⟩ לא תבחין בה זהר. מסירה הצמא, ומנחם המוח.

32 גַגַטרוֹם. דומה לשער גדי בנקודותיה. הנושאה יפחדו ממנו אויביו. ומלך קדמון היה נ⟨ו⟩שאה במלחמה וכל זמן שזאת האבן עליו מנצח; יום אחד שכחה ונהרג.

33 גַלַקְטִיטַש. קצת ירוקה, והירוק קצת כהה במראה. ואם תדקדק לראות—תארה כדשן עצי⟨ם⟩.

האשה הרוצה שיהיה לה חלב הרבה תכתש זאת האבן בנסיובי דחלבא ותשתה מיד אחר המרחץ, טרם תאכל דבר אחר. כטעם חלב גם מראיתה. ומי ששזר פתיל אחד מן צמר רחל, ינקוב זאת האבן, ויתלנה בצוארה באות⟨ו⟩ פתיל—ובא לה שפע חלב. ואם

1 מחיה: מרוה A   2 יקיא: emendation editor יהי MS   5 אם ישאנה emendation editor ומי שישאנה MS ‖ ימות emendation editor יכווה MS   13 במלחמה: emendation editor המלח MS   17 ששזר: emendation editor ששחק MS   18 ינקוב: emendation editor תרקוב MS

[67] Lat. gagatromeus is represented here as O. Fr. *gagatromé*, designating a stone that could not be identified; cf. Riddle, Marbode, no. 27, (gagatromeus): "Not mentioned in ancient sources other than Damigeron, there is no description given of this stone for identification purposes, other than that it is fawn-colored (capreole agrestia)".

[68] For Lat. *galactites*, 'galactite', cf. Riddle, *Marbode*, no. 42 (galactida): "is probably chalk or soft limestone, although it could refer to almost any soft, white stone or earth which can make a milky appearance in water".

[69] "whey" (*nasyuvei de ḥalba*); the Aramaic term features for instance in TB Pesaḥim 42a.

has a difficult parturition, he [the shepherd] should attach the stone to her belly, fastened with the mentioned thread. If someone wants his herd to [produce] much milk, he should wash this stone with pure water and salt and besprinkle his herd with it ere the sun rises: he will then have plenty of milk.

No evil will befall him who wears it, but if someone carries it in his mouth, it will confuse his mind. If one holds it against the sun, it will appear full with traversal lines and stripes.

34 ***Galictotea**:[70] [This stone] is green, like an emerald, but with [different] shades of white. Its virtue is unknown.

35 **Gelazias**:[71] [This stone] is entirely white, and its aspect is like that of ice. It cannot be heated by fire.

36 **Diadocode**:[72] It has the same aspect as beryl, it is pure on all its sides (facets). If someone throws it into a vessel with water, he can see as he pleases a species of demons, and they will answer whatever questions he may ask them. For there is nothing that coerces the demons to speak as well as does [this stone].

The scholars have therefore called it "holy", for if it is brought in contact with a corpse or with the cadaver of a bird or animal, it loses its force.

37 **Dionse**:[73] It is a black [stone] with red sparks. If one grinds/pulverizes it in water, he will perceive the odor of wine. Yet it takes away all odors of wine in the world, owing to the strength of its own odor. Ancient scholars found out by experience that whoever smells this stone immixed with water will not get drunk.

38 **Diamant**:[74] This [stone] by its power attracts iron. In the Holy Tongue [Hebrew] it is called *shamir*, as it is written: "as adamant, harder than flint".[75] Some of them have the size of a Greek bean. The large variety [...] is not large [...] and it somewhat tends towards the color of [rock-]crystal.[76]

---

70 This stone could not be identified.

71 *Gelazias* is M. Lat. for 'chalazia' (from Gr. for 'hailstone'), which is possibly a rough diamond or corundum; cf. Riddle, Marbode, no. 37, s.v. *gelatia*.

72 *Diadocode* is O. Fr. for 'diadocos' (from Gr. διάδοχος for 'substitute'); it was probably beryl or quartz; cf. Riddle, *Marbode*, no. 57.

היא מקשה ⟨י⟩שימנה על בטנה קשור בפתיל הנזכר. ומי שרוצה שיהיה לו חלב הרבה בעדרו ירחץ את [עדרו] זאת האבן במים זכי⟨ם⟩ ומלח, ובטרם יזרח השמש יזה המים בעדרו, אז יהיה לו שפע חלב.

ומי שנושאה לא יא⟨ו⟩נה לו רע, אך מי שנושאה בפיו יבלבל דעתו. האוחזה נגד השמש נרא⟨י⟩ת כולה מליאה בריחים ושירטוטים.

34 גַלִיקְטוֹטְיָא. ירוקה כעין אשמרלדא היא, אך מיני גונים לבנים בה. וכחה לא נודע.

35 גְלַקְצִיאַש. כולה לבנה, ועינה כעין הקרח. ולא יחם בעבור אש.

fol. 77a

36 דיאַדְקוֹדְא. עינה כעין בריל, | זכה בכל עבריה. מי שישליך אותה בכלי של מים יוכל לראות כחפצו מ⟨י⟩ן של השדים, והם יענו לו על כל שישאלם, כי אין דבר שיכריח השדים כמוה לדבר כל דבר.

על כן קראוה החכמ⟨ים⟩ קדושה, כי מי שיגע עליה מבשר מת או מנבלת עוף ובהמה תאבד כחה.

37 דְאוֹנִיש. שחורה ובה ניצוצות אדומות. הכותשה במים ימצא בה ריח יין. אבל גוזל כל ריח יין שבעולם מרוב ריחו. ונסו חכמי קדם כי לא יהיה שיכור ⟨מי⟩ שיריח מזאת האבן הממוסכת במים.

38 דִיאַמַנְט. זו מושכת הברזל בכחה. ובלשו⟨ן⟩ הקדש נקר⟨את⟩ שמיר והוא שכת⟨וב⟩ ״כשמיר חזק מצור״. יש מה⟨ם⟩ גדולה כפול יווני, והגדולה שבהם [...] אינה גדולה [...] וקצת נוטה לעין קרישטל.

---

2 ירחץ: emendation editor ינקב MS יכתת A ‖ יזרח: emendation editor יזרק MS 6 אשמרלדא: emendation editor אשמדאי הא MS 8 עבריה: emendation editor עבדיה MS 9 מ⟨י⟩ן של: מוצל A 10 לדבר: emendation editor ודבר MS 13 הכותשה: emendation editor הכותשר MS 16 מושכת emendation editor מנשכת MS

---

[73] *Dionise* is O. Fr. for 'dionysia'; the identification of this stone is uncertain; cf. Riddle, *Marbode*, no. 58.

[74] *Diamant* is O. Fr. for 'diamond'; cf. entry no. 1.

[75] Cf. Ez. 3:9.

[76] This statement is a virtual citation from entry no. 1, which also provides the reference, here implicit, to the loadstone.

Nothing can burst it, nor is it damaged by the power of fire. However, when they want to burst it so as to make two [stones] out of one, then they take the blood of a he-goat which is still warm, boil it, and steep [the stone] in that hot blood: this softens that which was hard. And subsequently [the stone] returns to its former [hard] state.

It is well-known that the diamond attracts iron. The diamond, owing to its strong power, takes the needle away from it [i.e. the loadstone]. Magicians make use of it. Whoever wears it when going to sleep will not have bad dreams, but [only] good ones; nor will he be harmed by poisonous reptiles.

It brings people back to their senses, it calms wrath and appeases lunacy. It keeps enemies away. [This stone] is mainly found amidst silver and gold. But since the power of this stone consumes silver and gold and destroys them, they[77] use to look for a robust iron called *ascir*[78] and set the stone in it. Its force [is active] when one carries it in his hand or in the left wing [of his garment]. [It is good for acquiring] wealth and courage. He who carries [it] continues to draw love [words missing or corrupted].[79] The power of this stone is perceptible especially when its color is like that of a polished (cut) crystal, tending somewhat towards [the color of] a lemon [*ethrog*] peel. That which has the color of peels that were [...] is very good.

39 ***Torquois** (*turquois*):[80] [This stone] is one of the varieties of the emeralds. But this variety is opaque white, somewhat leaning toward the green. The variety which is useful for eyesight and for modifying its surrounding [?] has green dots. The best [variety] has shades of colors, [called] *venes*[81] in the vernacular. If you find in it two black filaments, then it is very good.

If someone has intercourse with his wife, he will not corrupt his sperm as long as he wears [this stone]. But if someone wishes to cure his eyes [with this stone] he should not wear it when he sleeps with a woman, because she likes [...]. Its color is essentially median, like that of a garment that has been dyed with the color [called] *jaiet*.[82] It is good for hunters and warriors. Some people make an incision in the skin of their shoulder and sew the stone under the skin of their flesh. A wounded person will not die as long as he wears [this stone].

---

77 העולם perhaps in the sense of 'tout le monde', i.e. 'everyone'.

78 *Ascir* is Angl.-Nor. for 'steel'.

כל לא יפוצציה, ולא תנזק מכח אש. רק כשרוצים לנפצה ולעשות מאחת שתים יקחו דם תיש חם וירתיחוהו ויטבלוה באותו דם חם, אז ירך קשה. ואחרי כן תשוב לקדמ⟨ו⟩תה.

וידוע כי הדיאמנט מושך הברזל אליו. והדיאמנט מכחו הרב ממנה יגזול לה המחט. והמכשפים יעזרו ממנה. ואשר ישאנה עליו בשכבו לא יחלום חלום רע כי אם טוב, ולא חמת זחלי עפר יריע לו.

משיב דעת האדם, משכך חימה, משקיט שיגעון. מרחקת ש⟨ו⟩נאים. ועקר מושבה בכסף ובזהב, אך לפי שכח האבן מכלה הכסף והזהב ומשחיתו נהגו העולם לבקש ברזל חזק הנקר⟨א⟩ אַצִיר וישבצוה בו. וכחה לשאתה ביד או בזרוע או בכנף השמאלי. [...] לעושר ולגבור⟨ה⟩. ואותו הנושא שוב להמשיך אהב⟨ה⟩ המקבל עליו. ועיקר הכרת כח האבן ⟨ה⟩זאת כשהיא עין בדול⟨ח⟩ מלוטש, ועינו נוטה קצת לקליפת אתרוג. ואשר יש בו כעין קליפות שהיו [...] טוב מאד.

39 טוֹרְקְוִיש. מ⟨י⟩ן אחד ממינ⟨י⟩ אשמרלדא, אבל זה המין ממין לבן עב, וקצת נוטה לירוק. ויש נקדות ירוקות בה ממין אש⟨ר⟩ טובה למראית העין ולהפוך סביבותם. והטובה יש בה גווני⟨ם⟩ וינש בל⟨עז⟩. ואם תמצא בה שני חוטין שחורות טובה מאד.

המשמש עם אשתו כל זמן שהיא עליו לא ישחית זרעו. אבל מי שרוצה לרפא עיניו לא ישאנה עליו כאשר | fol. 77b ישכב עם אשה כי היא אוהבת ⟨...⟩. ועיקר מראיתה ממוצע, כעין בגד הנצבע מצבע גֵייטְא. טובה לאנשי ציד ולבעלי מלחמה. ויש מקרעין עורם על כתפם ותופרין א⟨ו⟩תה תחת עור בשרם, ולא ימות הנפצע כל זמן שהיא עליו.

---

2 תיש: emendation editor היש MS ‖ וירתיחוהו: emendation editor וירתיחוה MS 4 הדיאמנט: emendation editor ההיאמנט MS 10 הנושא: emendation editor הנתון MS 11 לקליפת: emendation editor כקליפת MS 14 לירוק: emendation editor לחוק MS 15 בה: emendation editor בם MS ‖ חוטין: emendation editor חיטין MS

---

79 The reading and translation of the last sentence is uncertain.

80 *Turquois* is O. Fr. for 'turquoise'. This stone does not feature in Marbode. The name "turquoise" dates from the Middle Ages when it was imported 'from the Turks'; it was probably described by earlier writers under other names; cf. Wyckoff, *Albertus Magnus*, p. 123.

81 Plural of Angl.-Nor. *vene*, 'vein'.

82 O. Fr. *jaiet*, 'jet'.

If you receive this stone [as a present] do not sell it, and if it is good, do not donate it: for it has the power to arouse hatred against the one who gives it away.

40 Topace:[83] It has two varieties. One is like [??]. The second [has the color of] a honeycomb. Many tried to cool boiling water with it. [In it] you see the inverted images of faces. For someone suffering from jaundice it is very beneficial to wear it. It is usually set in a ring of lead. One should wash it in wine three times a day, in the evening, morning and afternoon, and drink [the wine]. One should [also] write on parchment: ʾNQ, YWD(?), ṬRYP, PṬYR, ʾWGʿ, then wipe out what is written in wine, and drink this. The one who wears this stone will remove fear from his heart, and a dog will not wet his tongue at him (Ex. 11:7). If he loses something, it will be returned to him. It stops bleeding, eliminates nausea, and reduces a swelling.

41 Jaspe:[84] The best of all is the green [variety] which shines like a star. It is beneficial for fever and for dropsy. It strengthens the courage of him who wears it as long as he wears it in purity. It is beneficial for a woman having a difficult [childbirth] and against evil spirits. It is set principally in silver. The [jasper] that is green with red drops stops bleeding and gives success.

If one touches a man or a woman with any [jasper stone] that has red, black, or white hues, he can do with [or: to] them whatever he wishes. If one wraps it in wax, he will understand language[s] he does not know. Those that are speckled with different drops are very good. The sages said that if one turns in [different] directions a green [jasper] that is thin the drops are observed to move away from their [original] places. It prevents a man from begetting and a woman from conceiving. The one who wears it at sea will not drown.

42 Jaiet:[85] It is very light and black. It is of a pure blackness. If someone chafes it by rubbing, it raises [i.e. attracts] the straw. If someone wishes to set it ablaze he should wash the stone in water; it cannot then be quenched, except with olive oil.

---

[83] O. Fr. *topace* is 'topas', which, as described by Berakhyah, applies to two different stones: 1. a yellow or orange stone, our topaz but also other yellow stones like citrine quartz; 2. a stone that causes water to stop boiling and reflects objects like a concave mirror; i.e. hephaestites; Cf. Wyckoff, *Albertus Magnus*, p. 122; Riddle, *Marbode*, no. 13.

אם ינתן לך זאת האבן אל תמכרנה, ואם היא טובה אל תתנה, כי כחה לעורר שנאה על נותנה.

40 טוֹפַּסְא. שני מינין יש בה. האחד כפר רותם הב׳ יבישנוא [?], והשנית כנפת דבש. ונסו רבים להקר ממנה מים הרותחין. צורות פנים הפוכות תראה. ולמי שיש לו ירקון טובה מאד לשאתה. ועיקר מושבה בטבעת עופרת. וירחץ א⟨ו⟩תה ביין ג׳ פעמ⟨ים⟩ ביום ערב ובקר וצהרים וישתה. ויכתוב בקלף אחד אנק יוד טריף פטיר אוגע, וימחה הכתוב ביין וישתה. נושא זאת האבן יסי⟨ר⟩ מלבו פחד וכלב לא יחרץ לו לשונו. ואם אבד מאומה יחזירו לו. ומעצר⟨ת⟩ דם ומבטלת הקיא ומשפלת הנפח.

41 יַשְׁפֵא. הטובה מכולם היא הירוקה הזרחת כעין ככב. והיא טובה לקדחת ולחולי אדרופיק. מחזקת הנושאה בגבורה כל זמן שישאנה בנקיות. טובה למקשה ולרוח רעה. ועיקר מושבה בכסף. והירוקה אשר ימצא בה טיפות אדומות היא המעמדת הדם ומצלחת.

וכל אות⟨ה⟩ אשר גווני⟨ם⟩ בה אדום או שחור או לבן אם יגענו באיש או באשה יעשה מהם כחפצו. ואם יכרכנו בשעוה יבין לשון אשר לא ידע. והמנומרות מטיפות משונות טובה מאד. ואמ⟨רו⟩ החכמי⟨ם⟩ שהירוק⟨ה⟩ אם היא רקיקה, וכשפונים אתה לצדדים, יֵראו הטיפות כאשר יתנועעו ממקומן. מונעת האיש מלהוליד והאשה מלהתעבר. והנושאה בים לא יטבע.

42 יאייט. קל מאד ושחור לשחרות שבו זך. ומי שיחממו על ידי חיכוך מגביה הקש. ומי שרוצה להבעיר⟨ה⟩ ירחץ האבן במים אז לא יוכל לכבותו כי אם משמן זית.

5 ביין: emendation editor בשיניו MS   18 שיחממו: emendation editor שחיחממו MS ‖ חיכוך: emendation editor חיפות MS

[84] *Jaspe* is O. Fr. for 'jasper', which is cryptocrystalline silica. It possibly was a generic term, including other green stones—prase, chrysoprase and perhaps jade; cf. Wyckoff, *Albertus Magnus*, p. 100; Riddle, *Marbode*, no. 4.

[85] O. Fr. *jaiet* is 'jet', a bright black hydrocarbon, related to coal, cf. Riddle, *Marbode*, no. 18.

If someone fell ill with gout, which is between the skin and the flesh, he should wear [this stone] and touch [the affected spot] with it. The water in which the stone was washed strengthens loose teeth. If you want [to know whether a woman is virgin or not, you should] let her drink from the water in which the stone was washed: if she is no longer a virgin, she will urinate immediately, but if she does not, then she is certainly a virgin. The fumes of the stone are good for [the flux of] menstruating women. Wearing it is beneficial for epileptics and for chasing demons away. If someone suffers from an upset stomach he should drink from [water immixed with] the filings [scrapings] of the stone, and he will be cured. And if it is soaked in water for three days, it [i.e. the water in which it was immersed] cures the illnesses mentioned. Likewise, the water in which it has been soaked eases strong labour pains. The one who has a swelling should wear it.

43 **Gerachite:**[86] It is somewhat black. If someone first washes his[87] face and then puts it in his mouth, he can apprehend what his companion thinks of him. Whatever he may ask of people they will not deny him. With women he can do as he pleases.

It chases flies away. As for testing [the stone]: if one puts it in his mouth, he will perceive a taste like honey. Even if the stone is coated with milk or honey, it will chase the flies[88]. But when the stone is removed they[89] return to where they were.

44 **Gelazia:**[90]: It looks like hail which is called *gresil*[91] and is not larger than it, but ⟨…⟩. It is always cold and you cannot heat it [even] by pure fire. Whoever carries it in his mouth under his tongue will know some of the future occurrences. He who wears it need not fear fire. If someone wishes to know future occurrences, he should put it in his mouth at midday at the time of the New Moon, for such is its power. It belongs to the kinds [of stones] whose colors shine when looked at. It has circles around it.

---

86 *Gerachite* is O. Fr. for 'hieracitis'; the identity of this stone is uncertain. Wyckoff, *Albertus Magnus*, suggests that it is possibly arsenic ore, since it keeps insects away; however, the assertion of putting it in one's mouth argues against this, according to Riddle, *Marbode*, no. 30.

87 "his face": possibly to be corrected as: "this stone"; cf. A: "He who washes it in water".

88 "flies": "bees" A.

ומי שחלה מחלי גוטא שהיא בין עור לבשר ישאנו עליו ויגע בו. והמים אשר ירחצוה בהם יחזקו השנים המנענעות. ואם תרצה להשקות אשה ממי רח⟨י⟩צת האבן אם בעולה תשתין מיד ואם לא כן אז היא בתולה בודאי. והעשן מן האבן טוב להזיב נידות. ולשאתה טובה לנכפים | ולהבריח שדים. ומי שנהפך בטנו ישתה מגרידת האבן וירפא. ובמים fol. 78a ינתן ג׳ ימים לרפא החלאים שהזכרנו ומי שרייתה יתירו חבלי יולידה. והנפוח ישאנו.

43 יַרֲייטא. שחורה קצת. מי שרוחץ פניו תחילה וישים א⟨ו⟩תה בפיו יוכל להבין מה יחשב חבירו עליו. ומה שישאל מן האנשים לא ימנעו ממנ⟨ו⟩. ומן הנשים יעשה חפצו.

ומברחת הזב⟨ובים⟩. ובחינת האבן: הנותנה בפיו יטעם טעם דבש. ואפילו אם ימשחו האבן מחלב או מדבש אז יברחו ממנה הזבובים, ובעת יסירו ⟨אותה⟩ ישובו למקומן.

44 יילַצַא. היא כעין כפור שקורין גרזיל, ולא גדולה ממנו אלא ⟨...⟩. ולעולם היא קרה, ולא בצלולת אש תוכל לחממה. ומי שנושאה בפיו תחת לשונו יבין קצת העתידות. והנושאה לא יירא מאש. והרוצ⟨ה⟩ לדעת עתידות ישימנה בפיו לעת צהרים בחידוש הירח, כי כן כחה. והיא מן מיני גונים מבהיקין למראה העין. ועיגולים סביב לה.

3 בתולה: emendation editor בעולה MS 4 שנהפך (= A) emendation editor שנשפך MS || בטנו: emendation editor בענן MS 6 מי: emendation editor מה MS מי שרוחץ פניו (= אותה?): מי שרוחצה במים A 9 הזבובים: הדבורים A || ישובו למקומן: ישובו להלחם בחזקה A 10 שקורין: שיקורין MS 11 בצלולת: emendation editor בעלילת MS בצלולת אש cf. Pannier, Les plus anciens lapidaires français, p. 514, l. 1166: pur fu

[89] "they return to where they were": "they return to attack fiercely" A.

[90] *Gelazia* is M. Lat. for 'gelacia' (from Gr. for 'hailstone'); its identity is uncertain; Riddle, *Marbode*, no. 37, surmises that it is possibly a rough diamond or corundum.

[91] I.e., O. Fr. *gresil(le)*, 'hail'.

45 *Legnete:[92] There are two varieties [of this stone]: one is very pure and red, the other is purperlike. Each of them appears to the eye as clear, yet the eye is incapable of seeing through its entire thickness. If it is heated by the sun or by [rubbing it with] a garment, it lifts up [i.e. draws] the straw. Some call it "debris of carbuncle".[93] It is beneficial for evil spirits, and [it is beneficial] to fasten it to a man whose nose is bleeding. It is beneficial for [those who speak in] riddles, and is also [good] for lunatics to wear. When it is feared that a house may burn down because houses around it are on fire, one should place the stone vis-à-vis [the house], and the fire will retreat.

46 Ligurie:[94] It is yellow and has white and black spots. It attracts straw to it. It cures pain and the malady of gout, and makes the face of the head shiny (look healthy) again. Some call it *date*.[95]

47 *Medo (*medus*):[96] Many have tried its power for someone whose eyes have been blinded through an illness. One should take this stone, mix it [i.e. its powder] with the milk of a woman who gave birth to a male child, and apply it to his eyes until his eyesight is restored. And for gout one should immerse it in the milk of a goat and let [the patient] drink it [...]. For pain in the loins, one should rub them with the milk.

If someone wants to blind his enemy he should whet the stone on a red whetstone, [immersed] in clear water and rub some of it [i.e. the water with the stone particles] on the forehead of his enemy: he will instantly be blinded. If you let him drink from this water, he will vomit until he dies. The connoisseurs called it "black", but in its nature one also finds a greenish [shade]. When one wants to use [the stone] to do well, [he should employ] the greenish-white one; to do harm, [one should employ] the black one.

48 Perle:[97] It is white and it is called *margarite*.[98] It grows from a drop of dew, etc. It is good for [speaking well] in meetings and for pleasing [people].

---

[92] **Legnete* is a non-documented Romance form of Lat. *lignita*, 'lychnis'. The two varieties mentioned by Berakhyah are characterised by Pliny, *Natural History* 37.29.103, s.v. *lychnis*, as one having a purple and the other a scarlet sheen (trans. Eichholz), and are identified by Eichholz as violet-red and rose-red tourmaline respectively. The stone does not feature in Marbode.

45 לְינֵיטְא. שני מינים היא: האחת זכה ואדומה מאד, השנית כעין תכלת. וכל אחת צלולה לפי מראה העין אך לא תשלוט העין לראות כל עבי⟨ה⟩. ואם תחם משמש או מבגד תגבי⟨ה⟩ הקש. ויש קראוה פסולת קַרבוֹנְקלא. טובה לרוח רעה, ולקשור על איש אשר חוטמו זב דם. וטובה לחוד חדות, וגם למשגעים לנשוא. והבית אשר יראים ממנו פן יבע⟨ר⟩ בו האש כשבתים סביב לה מבערים, ישימו האבן מנגד, ויסוב האש לאחור.

46 לִיגוֹרֵיאַה. ירוקה ומנומרת מלבן ושחור. ומ⟨ו⟩שכת הקש אליה. והיא תרפא כאב וחולי גוטא, ומאירה פני הראש כמו שהיתה. ויש קוראים שמה דֵיטְא

47 מֵידו. רבים ניסו גבורת⟨ה⟩ לאשר עיניו נתעורו על ידי חולי. לקוח זאת האבן וימסכנה בחלב אשה אשר ילדה זכר, וימשח עיניו עד שוב אורו. ולגוטא יושם ⟨ב⟩חלב עז וישתה נסתיקומי [?]. ולכאב חלצים ימשחם מן החלב.

והרוצה לעוור אויבו ישחיז האבן במשחזת אדומה במים צלולים וימשח מהן מצח אויבו — מיד ⟨ית⟩עור. ואם תשקהו מן המים יקיא עד שימות. שחורה קראוה מכיר⟨י⟩ה, אבל בתולדתה תמצא ירקרקת. ובעת ירצו לפעול ממנה | להטיב: ירקרוקה לבנה; להרע: שחורה. fol. 78b

48 פֵּירְלְא. לבנה ונקר⟨את⟩ מרגריטא. מטיפת טל גידולה וכו׳. טובה לוועד ולשאת חן.

---

3 פסולת: emendation editor פסולק MS 4 וטובה: emendation editor ושבה MS 6 אליה: emendation editor אלא MS 7 הראש: emendation editor הרוח MS 9 אשה אשר: emendation editor אשר MS ‖ ילדה: emendation editor ילדת MS ‖ ולגוטא יושם: emendation editor ולגוטא הלב יושם MS 10 חלב עז: emendation editor עד חלב MS

---

[93] Cf. Pliny, *Natural History* 37.29.103: "remissiorem carbunculum"; also cf. Supplement B.

[94] O. Fr. *ligurie* is 'amber'; cf. Riddle, *Marbode*, no. 24.

[95] *Date* is Angl.-Nor. for 'urine'. One of the Greek names for amber was λυγκούϱιον, cf. Riddle, ibid.

[96] Lat. *medus* designates a stone that was probably a mixture of impure metallic sulphates; cf. Riddle, *Marbode*, no. 36.

[97] *Perle* is O. Fr. for 'pearl'.

[98] O. Fr. *margarite* is 'pearl'.

49 Pantera:[99] It is a kind of jasper, but its colors are green, black and red. It is somewhat dark, yet a luminescence issues from each color. If someone wears it and looks at it before sunrise, he will be feared by everyone and will be invincible in battle on that day.

50 Pedoretes:[100] [It is] white and its luminescence is somewhat like that of gold, but at a certain distance it does not shine. The nerves of the one who wears it will not contract. Therefore, it is said that it is beneficial for the nerves.

51 *Paitoros:[101] There are two varieties: one resembles red gold and the second is clear and white. It is beneficial for hemorrhoids, and cools boiling water.

52 *Peritora:[102] It is greenish and its brilliance is in the middle between that of the emerald and topaz. [They] set it in a silver ring and on the ring [they] write: ṬiBaQoṬ QWṬNY. It beneficial to wear it for *gote crampe*,[103] and he [the wearer] will be healed. These names are tried [as beneficial] for that illness also without [using] this stone.

53 Carboncle:[104] It burns like wood and burning coal. Neither darkness nor light darken its blaze. Some say that the ruby is an inferior kind of carbuncle. Both [stones] are equally good to reduce a swelling. To stop bleeding: if [the stone] has a hole it should be hung around the neck of the one who bleeds, above [or: applied to] the hair of his head, and it will stop the nosebleed. Someone who is feverish should wear it. He who wears it finds favor. Against the shining of the sun its luminiscence appears like that of a burning candle. The blaze it emits has no equal. Those that hail from the Orient are very good, their light shines in the darkness.[105]

---

99 Lat. *pantera* is 'panther stone', i.e. a variety of the opal; cf. Riddle, *Marbode*, no. 51.

100 *Pedoretes* is Angl.-Nor. for 'paedoros'; this stone, a kind of opal, and the exebenus feature in the *Cambridge Version of Marbode's Lapidary* as the only two real additions to the original Marbode; cf. Studer-Evans, *Anglo-Norman Lapidaries*, p. 154.

101 This stone could not be identified.

102 This stone could not be identified. The anonymous Hebrew Marbode translator possibly transcribes this stone as: PYRYDWN' (entry 63).

49 פַּנְטֵירַא. מן ישפה היא, אבל היא מן גוונים ירוק שחור ואדום. וקצת כהה, אבל זהר יצא מכל גון וגון. הנושאה ויביט עליה טרם זרוח השמש כל איש ירא מפניו, ואותו יום לא ינצח בו במלחמה.

50 פִּידוֹרַטַש. לבנה וקצת נוטה זהרה לזהב אבל לא תזרח רחוק ממנה. ⟨ה⟩נושאה לא יתקמטו גידיו. ע״כ אמרו כי היא טובה לגידים.

51 פַּיְיטוֹרוֹש. שני מיני⟨ם⟩: אחת דומה לזהב אדום, והשנית צלולה ולבנה. טובה לתחתונ⟨י⟩ות, ומים רותחין מצננת.

52 פְּרִיטוֹרַא. קצת ירוק⟨ה⟩ וזהרה ממוצע בין אשמרלדא ובין טופצא. ישבצוה לטבעת כסף, ועל הטבעת כתוב: טִיבַקוֹט קוטני. וטוב לשאתו לגוטא קרנפא. וגם אילו השמות בחונים לאותו חולי בלא זה האבן.

53 קַרְבוֹקְלא. בוער כעץ ⟨ו⟩גחל. לא חשך ולא אור יאפיל אורה. ויש אומ׳ כי רובין פסולת קרבוקלא. ושניהם טובים ושוים להשפיל נפח. להעמיד הדם: אם הוא נקוב יתלה בצואר המטפטף דם, על שער ראשו, יעמיד דם נחיריו. והנקדח ישאנו. ונושאה ⟨ימצא⟩ חן. וכנגד זריחת השמש יעלה זהרו כנר הדולק. והלהב היוצא ממנה אינה דומה ⟨לה⟩. והבאים מן אוריאנט טובים מאד. ובחשך יהלו אורם.

11 כעץ: emendation editor העץ MS 13 דם: emendation editor על MS ‖ על: emendation editor עד MS ‖ ונושאה: emendation editor ונושאת MS

103 O. Fr. *gote crampe* means 'gout and cramp that contracts the extremities'; also cf. below entry no. 64.

104 *Carboncle* is O. Fr. for 'carbuncle' and means in most medieval lapidaries any brilliant red, transparent gem. The Latin term carbunculus is a translation of Gr. ἄνθραξ, '(red hot) coal'; cf. Riddle, *Marbode*, no. 23; Wyckoff, *Albertus Magnus*, p. 77.

105 See Is. 13:10.

54 Coral:[106] Its aspect is red. Whoever wears it, will have his health invigorated, and he will not suffer from epilepsy: therefore, it is hung around the neck of boys. It is essential for the one who wears it that it be attached to his arm. If someone has fields, olive trees, or vineyards, it will increase their produce. [He who wears it] need not fear evil spirits. Galen said that it cures eye ache.[107] For toothache and a worn tooth one should rinse the stone in water and rub the teeth with that water.

There are two varieties of it: red and white. The red one, when it is pure and uniform, without too many holes and red, is very good. The white one, [even] when it has large holes, is [still] good. The red [variety] comforts the mind more than the white [variety]. If someone's heart burns [with longing] during the night, then, if it is a man, he should put the red [variety of the stone] in his mouth; and if it is a woman she [should do the same with] the white [stone]. It is beneficial to accelerate the delivery of a woman who has a difficult childbirth, and to stop the bleeding of a woman who suffers from an [excessive] menstrual flow. The one who wears the red one need not fear serpents nor reptiles. If someone pulverizes [this stone] in water and drinks it, he can hold serpents and scorpions in his hand and they will not harm him. If someone wears it in a battle he will prevail, and if he travels in a ship, he will not drown.

55 Colire:[108] Its color somewhat tends towards that of a sapphire and its shining tends to that of seawater. If someone wears it around his neck, he will not arouse the wrath and ire of the land's rulers.

56 *Cortolina (*cornoligne*):[109] It is thoroughly red, and the red is very dark: it basically looks like water that has been used to wash meat. Whoever wears it on his finger or around his neck will be little irascible and easy to appease. It stops bleeding anywhere [in the body], [namely,] after the blood on it has dried through the heat of the sun or the heat of fire. It is very beneficial to stop [excessive] menstrual bleeding of a woman.

---

[106] O. Fr. *coral* is our 'coral'; it was considered in antiquity and the Middle Ages as a sea-plant which turns into stone when touched by air; cf. Riddle, *Marbode*, no. 20.

[107] This statement could not be retrieved in Galen's works.

54 קוֹרַל. אדום למראיתו. הנושאה יחזק בבריאותו, ולא יהיה נכפה — על כן יתלוהו בצואר הנערים. והוא עיק⟨ר⟩ לנושאה שתהא קשורה על זרועו. למי שיש לו שדות, זיתים, כרמים — יוסיף בהצלחתם. ולא יירא מרוח רעה. ואמ⟨ר⟩ גליינוס שהיא תרפא כאב העינים. לכאב שן או שן בלויה ירחץ האבן במים, וישפשף בם השינים.

ושני מינים בהם אדום ולבן. האדום, בהיותו זך ושוה בלא רוב נקבים ואדום, טוב מאד. והלבן אם יש בו נקבי⟨ם⟩ גדולים אז טוב. והאדום מנחם המוח יותר מן הלבן. ומי שיבער לבו בקרבו בלילות — אם זכר ישים האדום | [fol. 79a] בפיו, והאשה הלבן. וטוב למקשה למהר לידתה, ולזבה לעצור דמיה. והנושא האדום לא יירא מנחשים ומזוחלי עפר. והכותת אותו במים ושותהו — יקח נחשים ועקרבים בידו — לא יזיקוהו. והנושאו במלחמה יגבר, וֹהה⟨ו⟩לך בספינה לא יטבע.

55 קוֹלֵירַא. עינה ⟨נוטה⟩ קצת לספיר, ונוטה למי הים בזריחתה. הנושא⟨ה⟩ בצוארו לא יבא לו אף וחימה מן מושלי הארץ.

56 קוֹרְטוֹלִינַא. אדומה כולה והאדום אופל מאד — ועיקר מראית⟨ה⟩ כמים שרחצו בו בשר. הנושאה באצבעו או בצוארו יהיה קשה לכעוס ונוח לרצות. מעמדת הדם בכל מקום שהוא, אחר אשר יבש הדם עליה מחום השמש או מחם האש. ולעצור זיבת האשה טוב מאד.

9 והכתת: והכח תת MS והכ תת scribal correction 10 יטבע: emendation editor יטביע MS

[108] Angl.-Nor. *colire* is 'collyria'; the identity of this stone, which does not feature in Marbode, but is listed in the *Alphabetical Lapidary* (cf. Supplement B-2), is uncertain.

[109] O. Fr. *cornoligne* is 'carnelian', i.e. a translucent, orange-to-red chalcedony; cf. Riddle, *Marbode*, no. 22; Wyckoff, *Albertus Magnus*, pp. 81–82.

57 Cristal:[110] Its whiteness is like the color of ice. There are three varieties of it. For a woman suffering from a difficult childbirth it is beneficial to attach it to her thigh, suspended by a woolen thread. In order to conceive: she should wash it and drink the water in which it was washed. To bring back the milk [of a breast-feeding woman]: pulverize it in honey, mix it, and let her drink it; the milk will be restored. If [her] breast milk ceased owing to a fever: pulverize [the stone] in water and let her drink it. If a breast-fed infant is ill and you are afraid to give him a medicine: pulverize it [in water] and let the nursing [mother] drink it; subsequently she should take the medicine susceptible to heal the infant, so that the infant will suck his medicine [with the milk].

58 Calcidonia:[111] There are three varieties [of this stone]: one is somewhat white, although not like crystal; one is somewhat yellow; and one is median between hyacinth and beryl. To appease quarrels, to bring people together, and for a woman suffering from a difficult childbirth it is beneficial to wear it on one's finger or around one's neck. The pierced [stone] one should hang on a hair of a donkey: he who wears it will be victorious, and need not fear water or fire. As long as one wears it, it should be preserved from being defiled through intercourse.

59 *Camahu (*camahieu*):[112] These stones mostly have projecting images. Those that come from an old quarry are the best: [they have] the image of a man stretching his arms and the area surrounding the image is beneath him. There are many varieties of this stone: one has white in the area [surrounding the image] and black beneath it; there is a red one; and there is a pale one. We can decide whether we have that stone only according to the area around the white.

In general, this stone preserves one's wealth, but if someone wears it in battle, he will be overpowered.

60 *Calcofine (*calcofone*):[113] It is black in its entirety. If you strike it with a hammer a sound will be heard far away, like when one strikes a bronze frying pan. The one who wears it without being defiled through cohabitation will always have a pleasant voice.

---

[110] *Cristal* is O. Fr. for '(rock) crystal', a clear, colorless quartz; cf. Riddle, *Marbode*, no. 41.

[111] *Calcidonia* is Lat. for 'chalcedony'; chalcedony today is a collective term for a waxy,

57 קְרִישְׁטַל. כעין הקרח ללובן. שלושה מינים ימצאו בה. טובה למקשה לקשור ביריכה תלוי בחוט צמר. ולהתעבר תרחצינה ותשתה מי רחיצתה. ולהשיב החלב: כתשיהו בדבש ומסכיהו ותשתה וישוב החלב. ואם אבדה חלבה מחמת קדחת: כתוש במים ותשתה. ואם הנער היונק חולה ואתה ירא להשקותו רפואה: כתשהו והשקה למינקת, ואחר תשתה הרפואה שיתכן לרפא הנער, ויינק הנער רפואתו.

58 קַלְצִידוֹנְיָא. שלשה מינים הם: יש לבנה קצת אך לא כקרישטל ויש צהובה קצת ויש ממוצעת בין אבן יציטא ובריל. טובה לשאת באצבע או ⟨בצואר⟩ לשכך לריב, ולוועד, ולמקשה. הנקובה יתלה בשער חמור הנושאה ינצח ולא יירא אש ומים. וצריך לשמרה מטינוף שגל בעוד⟨נה⟩ עליו.

59 קַמַהו. רוב מאילו האבני⟨ם⟩ צורותם בולטות. ואותם שהם ממחצב ישן הטובות: צורת אדם שוטח זרועיו והשדה סביב צורתו בשפלתו. זאת האבן על מינים הרבה: יש לבן על שדו ושחור בתחתיהן, ויש אדום, ויש כהה. לא יכולנו לשפוט [אם] יש לנו זאת האבן כי אם על פי השדה אשר סביב הלבן.

כלל זאת האבן תחזיק העושר ביד בעליו. אבל הנושאה במלחמה ינוצח.

fol. 79b 60 קַלְקוֹפִינָא. שחורת על פני כולה. ואם תכה עליה בפטיש ישמע | כקול למרחוק, כמו מכה על מחבת נחשת. הנושאה בלא טינוף שגל יהיה לו לעולם קול ערב.

3 אבדה חלבה: emendation editor אבדו חלבו MS   11 צורת: emendation editor צורות MS   12 שדו: emendation editor סודו MS

smooth quartz. In Antiquity it meant a variety of stones "from Chalcedon"; cf. Riddle, *Marbode*, no. 6.

[112] *Camahieu* is O. Fr. for 'cameo'; it is not treated in Marbode, but, e.g., in the Alphabetical Lapidary (cf. Supplement B-2).

[113] *Calcofone* is O. Fr. for 'chalcophonos' (from Gr. for 'brazen voice'), which is possibly phonolite, a volcanic rock like nepheline syenite with the presence of feldspathoids; cf. Riddle, *Marbode*, no. 53.

61 Robin:[114] We have [already] explained [this stone] in [our chapter] on the carbuncle.

62 Saphir:[115] It is divided into three [kinds]; [yet] the knowledge of its species is reserved for specialists only. One [species] is the *saphir jacint (jargunce saphire)*;[116] [in its color] it resembles the sky. The second [species] is the *wazzer saphir (jagunce evage)*[117] and it resembles water. The third is the *saphir orient*,[118] which is the most excellent one. On the top, its color tends to black, [but] if you look at its sides there is a white hue that issues from it, which is similar in its purity to the light of the sun. The virtue[s] of this stone are: it keeps its owner healthy and his limbs firm; he [the owner] will not easily be enticed to associate with fools; and[119] he who avoids jealousy will be protected by [it]. It sets free the one who has been shackled in iron chains and he will find grace. More than any other stone it is good for making peace. It alleviates external illnesses and it cools the fever of internal organs. It reduces a swelling and cures scurvy. It appeases headache and stops sweating; it is beneficial for the eyes. One should always, as long as the stone is with him, [keep it] from being defiled through intercourse.

Likewise with the *saphir jacint (jargunce saphire)*.[120] For someone suffering from insanity, one should administer the herb [called] "sage" (*Salvia officinalis*)[121] and the herb [called] *milfoil*[122] [as follows]: wash the *saphir*[123] in the juice of these herbs and let him drink this. To enlighten [i.e. improve] one's eyesight he should hang it around his neck. If someone is terrified by [frightening] thoughts, he should take red coral and white coral and asafetida (*Ferula asafoetida*) and dissolve [their powder?] in his saliva [lit. teeth water], [and drink this?]—he will then find relief from his thoughts. Put the *saphir jacint (jargunce saphire)*[124] on the chest of a sleeping woman and and she will confess all her secrets.

---

[114] Cf. entry no. 53 above.

[115] The *sapphirus* (O. Fr. *saphir*) of the ancients was lapis lazuli, a brilliant blue opaque of sodalite minerals. By the thirteenth century, however, *sapphirus* was beginning to mean transparent blue gems, especially blue corundum, our sapphire; cf. Wyckoff, *Albertus Magnus*, p. 115; Riddle, *Marbode*, no. 5.

[116] *Jargunce saphire* designated in O. Fr. a sapphire that resembles the jacinth.

[117] *Wazzer saphir* is, literally, 'watery sapphire' in O. Fr. / Middle High German; cf. *jagunce evage* in O. Fr.; also cf. Wyckoff, *Albertus Magnus*, p. 98, and n. 2: "water sapphire is iolite, a pale blue or violet variety of cordierite."

61 רוּבִּין. פירשנו עם קרבוקלא.

62 שפיר. נחלק לשלשה, וחכמת מינ⟨י⟩ה רק לבקיאים. האחד שפיר יַכֻּנְט והוא דומה לשמים. והשני וַוִשְׁר שפיר, דומה למים. והשלישי שפיר אוריאנט, הוא המעולה. עינו נוטה לצד שחרות על גבו, ובהביטך בו לצדדין עין לובן יצא ממנו כאור השמש לטהר. גבורת זאת האבן: מחזיק בעליו בבריאות ואיבריו בחוזק, ולא נקל להיות מפותה בין חברת פתאים, [הנשמר] מקנאה ישמרנו, ומתיר הנאסר בכבלי ברזל ונושא חן, ועל כל האבנים יועיל לעשות שלום, וחולי הגוף מבחוץ יקל ויקרר חום הקרב הפנימי, משפיל הנפח מרפא הגרב. משכך כאב ראש, מוציא זיעה, טוב לעינים. ותמיד ⟨ישמרנו⟩ מטנוף שגל ⟨כל⟩ עוד היות⟨ו⟩ עמו.

ועם שפיר יכֻּנְט: ליוצא מדעתו נות⟨ן⟩ עשב לשון אייל וע⟨שב⟩ מילפוייל ורחוץ השפי⟨ר⟩ במיץ העשבים וישתה. ולהאיר עיניו יתלהו בצוארו. והנבהל ממחשבות יקח קורל אדום וקורל לבן וחלתית וימחה כל זה במי שיניו—אז יקל ממחשבותיו. והשפיר יַכֻּנט שים על חזה אשה שהיא ישנה ותודה כל נעלמיה.

5 נקל: emendation editor בקל MS 6 הנשמר מקנאה ישמרנו: וישמרנו מקנאה A ‖ מקנאה ישמרנו: emendation editor מקנא הישמרנו MS 7 ויקרר: emendation editor ויח? MS 11 במיץ: emendation editor במין MS 13 נעלמיה: emendation editor עולמים MS

118 **saphir orient* is, literally, O. Fr. for 'sapphire of the orient'.

119 "and he who avoids jealousy will be protected by [it]": "It protects him against jealousy" A.

120 Cf. above in this entry.

121 Hebrew *leshon ha-ayyil* is a loan translation of the Arabic *lisān al-ayyil*, meaning sage.

122 *Milfoil* is O. Fr. for 'yarrow (Achillea millefolium)'.

123 Cf. above in this entry.

124 Cf. above in this entry.

The three species of the **jacant (jacinte)*[125] are [the following]. One is called **jacite (jacinte)*;[126] it is somewhat resembles the *topace*.[127] If you look at it closely, you will see that its light is neither dim (opaque) nor pale, but a mixture of both. It is a beneficial [stone]. The second [species] is white as the seawater and it is called **wazzer jacant (jagunce evage)*.[128] It is somewhat pale, similar to *cristal*,[129] but a little dark and clouded, so that you can see your image [reflected] in it. If you look at it carefully you imagine in it something similar to a violet flower. The third [species] is called **alestre* (?)[130] and it resembles the sky. Its virtue is to chase away despondency from the heart. He who wears it will not be fearful and no bad accident will befall him; and he will find favor in the eyes of his host.

Moreover, the *jacint*[131] which is called **jacite (jacinte)*[132] is divided into three [kinds]. One is granular, the second is all covered with bright spots, and the third is smooth. The one [with] bright spots is hot, the smooth one is neither cold nor hot, while the granular one does not endure fire [i.e. it is inflammable]. What they have in common is that their colors change with the weather: when the sky is clear, so are they; [when the sky is dark], they too are dark.

The **jagunce marine (jagunce evage)*[133] is beneficial in order to cool the heat [i.e. fever] of the one who carries it in his mouth. There is yet another kind [of jacinth], [namely] **jacint grenat (jagonce grenat)*,[134] which is red as blood. When set in gold, it has the power to cool the heat [fever] if one drinks the water in which it was washed.

63 **Solenite**:[135] A shine like a light issues from it. Its shining is thick (i.e. dim). Its hue is like honey, somewhat tending towards green. When the Moon waxes, it increases and when it wanes, it decreases. He who wears it will attract the love of the people. It is good for diarrhea and cough. It possesses this virtue [only] when the Moon waxes.

---

[125] *Jacinte* is O. Fr. for 'jacinth'; for the three species of the jacinth cf. Wyckoff, *Albertus Magnus*, p. 97, and Riddle, *Marbode*, no. 14.

[126] *Jacinte* is O. Fr. for 'jacinth'.

[127] *Topace* is O. Fr. for 'topaz'; cf. entry no. 40.

[128] For O. Fr. *jagunce evage*, cf. above in this entry.

[129] *Cristal* is O. Fr. for 'crystal'; cf. entry no. 57.

[130] This term could not be identified.

ושלשה מיני יַכִּנְט הם: אחת נקר⟨את⟩ יסיטא, דומה קצת לטופסא. אם תדקדק להביטה תראה אורה לא עב ולא כהה, אך ממוסך משני⟨הם⟩. והיא טובה. השנית לבנה כמי הים, והיא נק⟨ראת⟩ ושר יכנט. קצת כהה, דומה לקרישטל, אך חשו⟨כה⟩ קצת ומעוננת, שתוכל לראות בה צורתך. וכשתדקדק במבטה תראה בה כעין פרח ויאול. והשלישית נקרא עלישטרא. דומה לשמים, וכוחה שוה להבריח יגון הלב. הנושאה לא יפחד ולא יקרה ⟨לו⟩ פגע רע, וימצא חן בעיני האיש אשר יתארח עמו.

ועוד: יכנט הנקר⟨א⟩ יסיטא נחלק לשלשה. האחת גרעינין בה, השני בהרות בהרו⟨ת⟩, השלישי⟨ת⟩ חלקה. אותה שהיא בהרות חמה, והחלקה לא קרה ולא חמה, ובעלת הגרעינין לא תוכל לסבול האש. הצד השוה שבהם עם האויר יתחלפו מראיהן: כשהשמים בהירים גם הם כן, ⟨וכשהשמים חשוכים⟩ גם הם יחשכו. | fol. 80a והיגונצא מרינא טובה להקר החום לנושאה בפיו. עוד מין אחר, יכנט גרנט, אדום הוא כדם. ומשובצת בזהב כחה להקר החום לשתות מי רחיצתה.

63 שוֹלְנִיטֵי. נוגה כאור יוצא ממנה, וזריחתה עבה, ועינה כעין דבש, וקצת נוטה לירוק. ברבות הירח תרבה ובמיעוטה תמעט. הנושאה ימשוך אליו אהבת הבריות. וטובה לשלשולי⟨ם⟩ ולשיעולי⟨ם⟩. וכוחה ברבו⟨ת⟩ הירח.

---

3 ושר: emendation editor אשר MS 6 יפחד: emendation editor יבחד MS ‖ יקרה: יקרם יקרה but the first word was deleted by the scribe MS 7 יכנט: emendation editor יכיט MS 8 חלקה: emendation editor חלקם MS ‖ והחלקה: emendation editor והחלקם MS 9 האויר: emendation editor האייר MS 10 בהירים: emendation editor ברוצה MS 12 רחיצתה: emendation editor רחיצתם MS 13 ועינה: emendation editor ועינים

---

131 Cf. above in this entry.
132 Cf. above.
133 For *jagunce evage*, cf. above in this entry.
134 *Jagonce grenat* is literally 'garnet red jacinth' in O. Fr.
135 *Solenite* is Angl.-Nor. for 'moonstone'; it is used for transparent crystals of gypsum. Today the term moonstone is chatoyant or iridescent feldspar. Marbode possibly meant microline, a potash feldspar, which has a pale green color, sometines of gem quality; cf. Riddle, *Marbode*, no. 26.

64 Sardine:[136] Its [hue] is ⟨between⟩ reddish and red. It is very beautiful. However, it is has not the power of [...], yet it appeases bad dreams. The water in which it was washed is good for a burning [i.e. yearning] heart, and to remove fear. It also mitigates [lit. cools] the [evil] instinct and cures the illness of *crampe*[137] of the one who holds it in his hand.

65 *Sarde onique (*sardonice*):[138] It has two names, [corresponding] to the colors mixed in it, viz. white upon black, and black upon white. Its size is that of a bean, or a little bigger. Its hue is purple or like the incipient stage of brightening[139] plumage of a dove. When [the stone] has both colors [clearly distinguished] next to the black, then [the stone] is good: you then see the white, and above it red which is like blood.[140] He who wears it without defilement through intercourse need not fear iron [i.e. weapons]. The dark [dull] [stone] is better than the pure [brilliant] one. More about this [stone] can be found in the entry "onyx".

66 Serpentine:[141] Snake stone. It has many dots, and hues which are black, red and green, which you see shining. And there are [also] dark ones [i.e. hues which do not shine]. In these hues you can see something like the snake's circle. It is good for arousal [?].

67 Sadde:[142] This is a very precious [stone] similar to the stone [called] **prime (prame)*.[143] Many say that it is the best kind of the turquoise, which we described above.[144]

---

136 *Sardine* is O. Fr. for 'sard', a translucent reddish or yellowish-brown chalcedony, not so red as carnelian; cf. Wyckoff, *Albertus Magnus*, p. 116; Riddle, *Marbode*, no. 10.

137 *Crampe* is O. Fr. for 'cramp'.

138 *Sardonice* is O. Fr. for 'sardonix', a form of onyx, a variety of silica, which has alternating layers of sand (carnelian) and white, producing red and white bands; cf. Riddle, *Marbode*, no. 8. Steinschneider, *Lapidarien, ein culturgeschichtlicher Versuch*, p. 70, erroneously lists this entry as two different stones.

139 "brightening plumage of a dove" (*ẓihuv yonim*): For this expression cf. Mishnah Ḥullin 1:5.

140 The translation of this sentence is uncertain.

141 *Serpentine*, O. Fr. for 'snake stone'; this stone does not feature in Marbode. Nowadays it is considered to be a rock composed of chrysotile and antigorite often in layers with or without other minerals having usually a dull green color often with a spotted or mottled appearance or a red or brownish hue due to the presence of iron; cf. *Webster's Third New*

64 שַׁרְדִּינְא. ⟨בין⟩ אדומה בין אדמדם, ויפת ⟨מראה⟩ מאד. אך אין בה כח שוכני [?] הטוב, אך חלומות רעים משקטת. ומי רחיצתה טוב ללב בוער, ולהסיר ⟨הפחד⟩. ומקררת יצר ומרפא חולי קרנפא לנושאה בידו.

65 שַׁרְדַא אוֹנִיקַא. בית שמות יש לה, כאשר גוונים יתערבו לה לבן על השחור ושחור על הלבן. ומדתה כפול ויותר מעט. ועינה פורפירא או כתחילת ציהוב יונים. בהיות גווניהם יחד אצל שחרות טובה תראה הלובן ומעל לו אדום כדם. הנושאה בלא טנ⟨ו⟩ף שגל לא ירא מברזל. והאפיל⟨ה⟩ טובה מן הזכה. ועוד בכך עליה בערך אוניקא.

66 שרפנטינא. אבן נחש. יש בה נקודות הרבה, ועינייני גוונים שחורים אדומים וירוקים, זורחי⟨ם⟩ למראה העין. ויש חשוכים. וכעין עיגול הנחש תוכל לראות בגוונים. טובה להער.

67 שדד. יקרה מאד ודומה לאבן פרימא. ורבים אומ⟨רים⟩ שהיא הטובה שבטורקוייש שכתבנו לעיל.

2 ולהסיר ⟨הפחד⟩: cf. Arnoldus Saxo (ed. Stange), p. 74: et pellit timorem   5 ומדתה emendation editor ומתנה MS   8 שרפנטינא: emendation editor פרפנשינא MS ‖ הרבה: emendation editor הדבר MS ‖ וירוקים: emendation editor וירוקיה MS   11 שדד: emendation editor שרד MS

International Dictionary, p. 2074. The stone allegedly received its name because of its protective powers against snakes' bites; cf. the poem attributed to Orpheus and said to have been written in the 4th century AD (http://www.cst.cmich.edu/users/dietr1rv/serpentine.htm):

> No more the trailing serpent's tooth to fear.
> Let him who by the dragon's fang hath bled,
> On the dire wound Serpentine powdered spread,
> And in the stone his sure reliance place,
> For wounds inflicted by the reptile race.

[142] *Sadde* is O. Fr. for 'barnacle shells'; cf. Marbode no. 35.

[143] *Prame* is O. Fr. for 'prase', a green stone.

[144] Cf. entry 39 above.

68 Taršiš:[145] Its color is like that of froth on water. It is useful for extracting worms from the body. Proceed as follows: Rub the stone with olive oil [and put it on] his [the patient's] belly. [...] The one that is called *ceraune*[146] and it is beneficial (?). It is useful to improve dreams. It is set in a tin ring.

69 Donkey-stone:[147] It is found in the brain of a donkey: white, greenish and porous as a sponge, and its color is pale. It is good for a woman in difficult childbirth to have it on her, touching her belly. It is [also] good for someone who took a fatal poison: [one should] grind the stone in water and have him [the patient] drink it; [idem for] someone bitten by a reptile.

70 Tortoise-stone:[148] It is beneficial for someone partaking of a meal with his foes, so that they may not feed him with a deadly poison. Its description is: it is pale and somewhat porous underneath. Some say that it increases love and preserves wealth.

71 Cilidonia:[149] It can be found in a bird called **aradnela* (*arondele*),[150] [namely] in its intestines or in the nest of its fledglings. Two kinds [of this stone] exist: one is entirely black or has black spots; and there is a red one. The red one is very beneficial for those who have an epileptic [fit] with the New Moon; it pleases and greatly alleviates the malady of the stone.[151] The one who wears it, should wrap it in a white, clean linen garment and put that garment in a honey-colored pouch, and hang it on his left side. Then he will find favor in the eyes of all those who see him. With the black [variety] one should proceed in the same way.

[145] Taršiš features as one of the stones featuring in the breastplate (Ex. 28.20); it is possibly identical with the mineral known today as "aquamarine"; cf. entry "Precious Stones and Jewelry", *Encyclopaedia Judaica*, vol. 13, col. 1010.

[146] O. Fr. *ceraune* is 'ceraunius, thunder-stone'; cf. Cambridge Version of Marbode's Lapidary, no. 27 (ed. Studer-Evans); see entry 72 below.

[147] This stone could not be identified. The entry is probably a later addition as it is not part of the alphabetical arrangement of the text.

68 תרשיש. מראיה כקצף על פני מים. מועלת להוציא תולעים מן הגוף. וכה תעשה: משח האבן בשמן זית על בטנו. הנקרא צירוניא ויועיל. וטובה להטיב החלומות. ומושבה בטבעת בדיל.

69 אבן של חמור. במוח ראש החמור תמצא לבנה ירקרקת ומנוקבת כמו ספוג ועינה כהה. טובה למקשה להיות עליה להגיע אל בטנה. וטובה לאשר אכל סם המות לגרד את האבן במים להשקותו; ולנשוך מזוחלי עפר.

70 אבן הצב. טובה לאוכל בין שונאיו פן יאכילוהו סם המות. ותארה: כהה וחלולה קצת מתחת. ויש אומ⟨רים⟩ כי תוסיף אהבה ותשמור העושר.

fol. 80b

71 צִילִידוֹנְיָא. תמצאינו בעוף ששמו אַרְדנלא במעיו או בקן גוזליו. ושני מינים ימצאו בם האחת שחורה כולה או כתמים שחורים בה ויש אדומה. האדומה טובה מאד לנכפים בחידוש הירח ונושא⟨ת⟩ חן וחולי אבן תקל מאד. אך צריך הנושאה שיקשרנה בבגד פשתן לבן זך ונקי ויתן אותו בגד בכיס צבוע מצבע כטיפת דבש ואצל צלע שמאלית יתלנה. אז ימצא חן בעיני כל רואיו. והשחורה גם היא כמשפט הזה יעשה לה.

---

2 צירוניא: The second yud has been added by the scribe above the line 9 אַרְדנלא: ארונדלא corrected in the MS 11 אבן: ישן A 12 בכיס emendation editor בפיס MS 13 ימצא: emendation editor יבוא MS || חן: בעיניו add. MS

---

148 Tortoise-stone: The name of this stone is the same as "chelonia-chelonis" (Greek for "tortoise") in Pliny, *Natural History* 37.56.155, and "chelonites" in Marbode, ed. Riddle, no. 39. However, its virtues are different from those in Pliny and Marbode. The entry is possibly a later addition.

149 *Cilidonia* is M. Lat. for 'chelidony', i.e. a red, white, or black stone found in the stomach of a swallow, according to the ancient and medieval tradition; cf. Riddle, *Marbode*, no. 17.

150 O. Fr. *arondel(l)e* is '(little) swallow'.

151 I.e. stones in the kidney or bladder. A has: "chronic disease".

He who hangs it on him will not suffer from fever, and will not be affected by strife, for it soothes even the wrath of the king. He who washes his eyes with water in which the stone had been immersed, his eyes will be cured him from many diseases. It is verily known that if one blinds one of the fledglings of the swallow with a peg of the tree called *cipres*,[152] and after three days goes to see it, his eyesight will be as before. It is well known that the stone grows in the intestines or gizzard of that bird, or [is found] in the nest with the fledglings. If one blinds one of its fledglings ⟨...⟩, the mother will cure it with a herb. The head of the cured bird is beneficial for the eyes. Someone who suffers from a fever or from [superfluous] humor should carry it on him; likewise someone who wants to undertake and finish a major accomplishment.

72 ***Ceriaun (ceraune):**[153] It is called "thunderstone" because it comes down with the thunder. Its color is somewhat similar to crystal. Wherever it is, neither lightning nor thunder will cause harm. If it is carried in a ship, the latter will not sink or wrack, and the wind will not harm it. It is beneficial for meetings, and for becoming victorious in battle. He who wears it while lying down, will have good dreams. There are two varieties: one is similar to a flame and the other looks like ice.

This is the end of [the treatise] *The Virtues of the Stones*

---

152 *Cipres* is O. Fr. for 'cypress (Cypressus sempervirens)'.

153 O. Fr. *ceraune* is 'thunder-stone'. The identity of this stone is uncertain. Marbode probably refers to crystals present after a washing rainstorm and to meteorites; cf. Riddle, *Marbode*, no. 28.

ומי שתולה זאת האבן עליו לא יארע לו קדחת ולא יחוש למריבו⟨ת⟩ כי גם חמת המלך תשכך. והרוחץ עיניו במים שתנתן בם ירפאו מחלאים רבים. וידוע באמת כי אם יתעוור האחד מאפרוחי ארונדל ביתד של עץ הנק׳ צִיפּרַש ואחר ג׳ ימים ילך לראותו אז יאורו עיניו כקדמתו. בידוע כי אותו ⟨עוף⟩ מגדל האבן במעיו או בקורקבן או הוא בקן עם הגוזלות. והמעוור אחד מאפרוחיו ומפרצו(?) האם תרפאנו בעשב. וראש העוף הנרפא טוב לעינים. והנקדח או בעל ליחה שישאנה עליו או מי שירצה להתחיל ולגמור דבר גדול.

72 צֵירִיאוֹן. יש קוראי⟨ם⟩ לה אבן ברק כי נופלת עם הברק. מראיתה דומ⟨ה⟩ קצת לקרישטל. בכל מקום שהיא לא יזיק שם ברק ורעם. ואם היא בספינה לא תטבע ולא תשב⟨ר⟩, ורו⟨ח⟩ לא יזיקנה. וטובה לוועד; ולנצח ⟨ב⟩מלחמה. והנ⟨ו⟩שאה בשכבו יחלום חלום טוב. ושני מינים הם: האחת דומה לשלהבת, והשינית דומה לקרח.

סליק כח של אבנים.

---

2 ירפאו: ולא יחוש למריבות added and then deleted by the scribe   6 שישאנה: emendation editor שאני MS   8 ברק: emendation editor ברד MS ‖ הברק: emendation editor הברד MS   11 לשלהבת: emendation editor לשליימה MS

SUPPLEMENT A

COMPARATIVE TABLE

Berakhyah	Anonymous Hebrew translator of Marbode
2. אקטץ. הנהר אשר יוציאו זה ממנו נקרא בו, והוא בארץ שְׁזִילְא. שחור הוא כעורב וסביבה עוגל לבן אשר זר לו סבי⟨ב⟩. וכמה מיני צורו⟨ת⟩ נמצאים בה בלא מעשה ידי אדם. ומלכים קדמונים הורגלו לנשאה כי כח גדול יש לה במלחמה, וגם כי חותמם ממנה ולא חלו בה ידים לפתח פתוחה. ובארץ קַרֵיטְא נמצא אבן קוֹרָל הדומה להם, אך כי יש בה גוונים דומים לזהב. והוא יקר מאד, וקראוהו סגולת מלכים. הנושאוֹ לא יירא מנחש ועקרב, ולא מכל זוחלי עפר. יש בהם מצורות ענפי יער, ויש בה⟨ם⟩ צורתם חיות מדבריות, יש מהם משיבים נפש שוקקה למים, יש מהם מאירות עינים כהות, יש מריחות מהם ריח טוב כבושם בוער באש. הנושאה ימצא חן בעיני רואיו. ויתנחם מצערו כל נושאה בלב שלם ובדעת נכונה.	2. אַקַטְא. על שם הנהר הנמצאת בתוכו הנקרא אַקַטְא בארץ שֵׁזִילְיָיא. שחורה כעורב או כגחל וסביבותיה עוגל לובן אשר זיר לה סביב והיא מתחלקת לכמה גוונים מן צורות בתוכה בלא מעשה ידי אדם. וזאת האבן מצאנו כי מלכים קדמונים נשאוה לפי שחותמה ממנה בלא פעולה. ובארץ קריטא נמצאת אבן ה⟨נ⟩קראת קורל וכדמותה אך יש בו גוונים דומין לזהב. והוא יקר מאד וקראוהו סגולת מלכים כי באוצרם יאצרוהו. והנושאו לא יירא מחמת נחש וארס עקרב. וְבאִינְדְא מוצאים אותם ובהם נמצא חיות מדבריות. ויש בהם צורת ענפי יער. ויש משיבים נפש שוקקה למים. ויש מאירות עינים כיהות. ויש מהם מריחות ריח כמור בוער באש. והנושא אקטא ישא חן בעיני כל רואיו בוקר וערב יתנחם מצערו ומאד טוב לנושאה בלב שלם ונבון.
2. Acates: it is so called after a river from which it is won, and which is in the land of Sicily. It is black as a raven and has a white circle around it, encircled by a brim. Embedded in it are various kinds of shapes, which are not man-made. Kings of old used to wear it, because it is very powerful in battle and also because their seal was made of it, [showing that] no hands interfered with it to engrave it. In the land of Crete the coral stone is found, which resembles it [lit. them], except that it has hues similar to gold. It is very precious and is called the treasure [*segullah*] of kings. He who wears it need not fear nor serpent, nor scorpion, nor any reptile.	2. ʾaQaṬəʾ (*agate*): It is [called] after the name of a river called "ʾaQaṬəʾ", [which is] in the land of Sicily. It is black as a raven or as a coal, and has a white circle around it, encircled by a brim. It has several colory shapes, like the skin of a panther, embedded in it, which are not man-made. We found that ancient kings wore it because their seal was made of it, without any human interference. In the land of Crete a stone is found which is called "coral"; it resembles it, except that it has hues similar to gold. It is very precious and is called the treasure [*segullah*] of kings because it was kept in their treasury. He who wears it need not fear nor serpent, nor scorpion. In India one can find them while they have the shape of desert creatures in them.

Some have forms like that of boughs from woods, some have the form of desert creatures. Some satiate the soul longing for water, some afford light to dim eyes. Some of them emanate an odor that is as good as spices burning in the fire. The one who wears it pleases those who see him. Everyone who wears it with a whole heart and with true understanding will be comforted of his grief.

Some have shapes like that of boughs from woods in them. Some satiate the soul longing for water, some afford light to dim eyes. Some of them emanate an odor like that of myrrh burning in the fire. The one who wears the agate pleases all those who see him in the morning and evening (all day long); he will be comforted of his grief; it is especially good for someone who wears it a with whole and wise heart.

---

3. אַלֵיקְטוּיְינָא. אחר שלש שנים לסירוס התרנגול זאת האבן ששמה בו צומחת קרוב לקורקבן. וכל המינים לא ישוו בה אם נלקחת מן התרנגול בעתה, שזהו אחר שבע שנים אחר סירוסו, היא נגמרת כולה. הגדולה כעין מיני קיטנית שקורי⟨ם⟩ פיבא. ותארה לבן כעין קרישטל אך לא מכל וכל. ויש תרנגול שנמצאת במעיו, ויש סביב הירך, ויש על⟨...⟩הנושאה ינצח אויביו במלחמה, ועל כן מלכים קדמונים נשאוה. מחזקת העושר בחזקתו, והסחרים מצליחים ושבים לביתם בנשא אותה. המשימה לא צמא, והנשאה בין שיניו ימצא חן בעיני כל. מעירה התאוה, ממלאה המוח, וטובה למקשה לילד. והגבירות ישאוה למצא חן בעיני האנשים, ועוצם גבורתה לנשאה בפיו.

3. אֱלִיקַטוּיינא הוא הנקרא בלשון אשכנז קפשטין. אחר שלש שנים לסירוס התרנגול צומחת בקרבו קרוב לקורקבן יְוזֵיר(?) בלע׳. וכל חפצים לא ישוו בה אם נלקחה בעתה מן התרנגול והוא אחר שבע שנים לסירוס התרנגול כי אז היא ⟨נגמרת⟩ כולה. וגדולה כמו פול פֵּיבְא ועינה כעין קרישטל ללובן.

והנושאה לא ינוצח במלחמה ומלכים קדמונים בטחו עליה לנצח⟨ב⟩מלחמתם. והנושאה בשעבוד? ישוב לביתו. והמשימה בפיו לא יצמא ואשר ישאנה בין שיניו ישא חן בעיני כל רואיו. ומעירה התאוה וממלאה המוח וטובה למקשה לילד. והגבירות ישאוה לשאת חן בעיני בעליהן ועוצם גבורתו לנושאה בפיו.

3. Alectuene (*alectoire*): Three years after the castration of the cock this stone, which is named after it, grows close to its stomach. No species of stone is comparable to it if it is removed from the cock at the right time, which is seven years after the castration, [at which time] it is full-grown. The largest one resembles a bean which is called "feve." Its aspect is white, like crystal, but not through and through. In some cocks it is found in the intestines, in others around the hip, in others in ⟨...⟩.

Whoever carries it defeats his enemies in war, wherefore ancient kings used to wear it. Possessing it increases wealth, and merchants who carry it are successful and return home. Whoever wears it will not be thirsty, and who carries it between his teeth will please everyone. It arouses sexual desire, fills the brain, and is beneficial for a woman in hard labour. Ladies wear it to please men, and it is extremely powerful when one carries it in his mouth.

3. ʾaLiYQaṭWoYYNʾ (*alectoire*): This is [the stone] called "Kapstein" in German. Three years after the castration of the cock this stone grows inside it, close to its gizzard [which is called] "YWZYR" in Romance. Nothing is comparable to it if it is removed from the cock at the right time, which is seven years after the castration of the cock, for then it is full-grown. The [largest] one resembles a bean [which is called] "feve;" it gives women lust [to sleep with men].

Whoever carries it suffers no defeat in war; ancient kings relied on it for gaining the victory in their wars. He who wears it in captivity will return home; he who carries it in his mouth will not be thirsty, and who carries it between his teeth will please all those who see him. It arouses sexual desire, fills the brain, and is beneficial for a woman in hard labour. Ladies wear it to please men, and it is extremely powerful when one carries it in his mouth.

17. אִירוֹנְא. זאת האבן באה מים סוף וכאבן קרישטל מראה. והערביים א⟨ו⟩הבין אותה ומביאין אותה מן הים. ולעולם נמצאו בה ששה קצוות. מי שיאחז בה בבית נגד זריחת השמ⟨ש⟩ מְנַגֵּהַ נגדו יכול לראות בקירות הבית כמה גוונים, כמראה הקשת אשר בשמים. כחה לתת [ניצחון] במלחמה, ובעבור גודל כוחה קראוה אירונא (= איריש?).	47. אירוגא היא אבן הבאה מים סוף. וערביים מביאין אותה וכקרישטל מראיה. ולה קצוות. ומי שיאחזנה בבית נגד זריחת ⟨השמש⟩ מנוגה נגדה תוכל לראותה בקירות הבית וכל מראות גוונים שלה.
17. *Irone (*iris*): This stone hails from the Red Sea. Its colour is like that of the crystal. The Arabs love [this stone] and fetch it from the sea. It always has six sides (hexagonal). If one holds it up in a house against the rising sun, [i.e. with the sun] shining opposite to him, he will see on the walls of the house a few colours, like those of the rainbow in the sky. Its virtue is to give [victory] in war, and on account of its great virtue it has been called "ironye".	47. ʾYRWGʾ (*iris*): This is a stone that hails from the Red Sea. The Arabs fetch it [from the sea]. Its colour is like that of the crystal. It has [six] sides. If one holds it up in a house against the rising sun, [i.e. with the sun] shining opposite to him, he will see it and all its different colours on the walls of the house.
18. אַנְדְּרוֹ דְּרַגַּצָא. בחול של שפת ים תמצא מראיתה ככסף מזוקק וקשה כאבני אאימנט וטובה לשכך אף וחימה.	48. אנרוזרגמא. היא אבן הנמצאת בחול אשר על ים סוף והיא מרובעת ומראיתה ככסף מזוקק וקשה כאבן איימנט ומכשפים קדמונים אמרו מי שחמתו בערה ונשא זאת האבן ישכך חמתו.
18. *Andro dragaza (*androdragma*): You find it in the sand on the seashore. Its appearance is like that of refined silver. It is as hard as the diamant. It is good to calm wrath and anger.	48. ʾNRWZRGMʾ (*androdragma*): This is a stone that is found in the sand of the strand of the Red Sea. It is quadrangular and its appearance is like that of refined silver and it is as hard as the diamant. Ancient magicians said that if someone whose anger burns [within him] carries this stone, his anger will abate.
19. אופטליאש. זאת האבן כחה לרפ⟨אות⟩ העין במי רחיצתה. והגנבים בעת יחתרו בתים ישאוה, לפי שהיא תאיר להם בחשך ויראו כל אשר בבית, ואותם שבבית לא יראום ולא ירגישו בם, ויקחו כל חפצם.	49. אוּפְּטַלְיְאשׁ. זאת האבן מוציאה כאב העינים בכחה. והגנבים ישאוה עמם בלכתם לגנוב כי מי אשר ישאנה יראה בכל מקום שילך כמו בצהרים. והאנשים אשר ימצאו שם לא יראו כלל ויוכל לקחת הון כחפצו.
19. *Optallies (*optallie*): This stone has the power to heal the eye with the water in which it has been washed. Thieves wear it while they search houses, for it affords them light in the dark and they see all that is in the house. But those who are in the house do not see or notice them. The [thieves] thus take whatever they wish.	49. ʾWPṬaLiʾuŠ (*optallie*): This stone has the power to alleviate pain in the eyes. Thieves wear it when they go stealing for he who wears it can see wherever he goes as if it was midday. But those who are there do not see anything at all, so that he can take as much property as he wants.

20. אַבְשִׁיטַא. שחורה היא, וגוונים אדומות יש בה. והיא שוקלת יותר מכל דבר שגדול כמוה. מי שיחם אותה באש פעם אחת תהיה חמה כל שבעת הימים.

20. Absite: It is black with red [veins]. It weighs more than anything of the same size. If someone heats it in fire a single time, it remains hot for seven whole days.

52. אבשיטא. שחורה היא וגוונים אדומות יש בה. והיא שוקלת יותר מדבר גדול ממנה ואם אבן או ברזל או עץ. מי שיחם אותה יהיה חם ז׳ ימים.

52. ʾBSYṬʾ (*absite*): It is black with red [veins]. It weighs more than anything larger than it, whether it is [from] stone, iron or wood. If someone heats it, it remains hot for seven days.

---

27. אַמַאֻונְטְש. ממוצעת בין שחו⟨ר⟩ לאדום, מנחמת הגוף. וכאשר תער⟨ב⟩ עפרה עם לובן ביצה תקל חולי עפעפים ומאירה העינים. טוב מאד לשתות למי שאכל סם המות. והיא תפוצץ האבן אשר במקוה השתן.

27. *Amauntes (*amiantus*(?)): Its [color] is intermediate between black and red. It relieves the body. If you mix its powder with egg white, it alleviates the illness of the eyelids and enlightens the eyes [i.e. improves eyesight].
It is very good to drink for someone who ingested a deadly poison. It pulverizes the stone in the urinary bladder.

67. אמאונטש. מנחמת הגוף וכאשר תערב עפרה עם לובן ביצה תקל חולי העפעפים ומאירה העינים. וטוב למי שמקיא דם ומעצרת זיבות ושילשול ועם יין טוב תשתה אותו למי שאכל סם המות ולשבר האבן במקוות השתן הוא טוב.

67. ʾMʾWNṬŠ (*amiantus*(?)): It relieves the body. If you mix its powder with egg white, it alleviates the illness of the eyelids and enlightens the eyes [i.e. improves eyesight]. It is benefical for someone who brings up blood and stops [excessive] menstrual flow and diarrhea. If you administer it with wine it is beneficial for someone who ingested a deadly poison. It is [also] good for pulverizing the stone in the urinary bladder.

---

32. גַגַטרוֹם. דומה לשער גדי בנקודותיה. הנושאה יפחדו ממנו אויביו. ומלך קדמון היה נ⟨ו⟩שאה במלחמה וכל זמן שזאת האבן עליו ⟨היה⟩ מנצח; יום אחד שכחה ונהרג.

32. Gagatromé: By its spots it resembles the hair [pelt] of a lamb. The one who wears it will be dreaded by his enemies. An ancient king used to wear it in battle, and was victorious as long as he wore it; one day he forgot [to wear] it and was killed.

26. גַנְטֵרוּס. היא דומה לשער גדי. ומי שישאנה עליו אויביו יברחו ממנו. ומלך אחד נשאה בהלחמו עם אויביו ונצחם, יום אחד שכחה ונהרג הוא.

26. GaNṬeRWuS (*gagatromeus*): It resembles the hair [pelt] of a lamb. If someone wears it, his enemies will flee for him. A king [used to] wear it when he fought against his enemies and to defeat them. One day he forgot [to wear] it and he was killed.

33. גַלַקְטִיטַש. קצת ירוקה, והירוק קצת כהה במראה. ואם תדקדק לראות—תארה כדשן עצי⟨ם⟩.
האשה הרוצה שיהיה לה חלב הרבה תכתש זאת האבן בנסיובי דחלבא ותשתה מיד אחר המרחץ, טרם תאכל דבר אחר. כטעם חלב גם מראיתה. ומי ששזר פתיל אחד מן צמר רחל, ינקוב זאת האבן, ויתלנה בצוארה באות⟨ו⟩ פתיל—ובא לה שפע חלב. ואם היא מקשה ⟨י⟩שימנה על בטנה קשור בפתיל הנזכר. ומי שרוצה שיהיה לו חלב הרבה בעדרו ירחץ את [עדרו] זאת האבן במים זכי⟨ם⟩ ומלח, ובטרם יזרח השמש יזה המים בעדרו, אז יהיה לו שפע חלב. ומי שנושאה לא יא⟨ו⟩נה לו רע, אך מי שנושאה בפיו יבלבל דעתו. האוחזה נגד השמש נרא⟨י⟩ת כולה מליאה בריחים ושירטוטים.

40. גלטירא. ב׳ מינין הן ובשני נהרות ימצאם האחד נילוס והשיני אין ליאוש.
ואשה שרוצה להרבות חלבה יכתתנה וישתהו אחר המרחץ מיד טרם תאכל.
ומי שתקח מעט צמר מרחל ויטוה פתיל אחד ויקוב זה האבן וישים הפתיל בתוכה ויתלנה בצוארה ואז יהיה לה שפע חלב. וכשתהיה מקשה לילד תשימנה על בטנה אך יהיה קשור באותו פתיל שהזכרתי. ומי שרוצה שיהיה לעדרו חלב הרבה יכתת זה האבן במים זכים ומלה וטרם יזרח השמש יזה מן המים על עדרו ויהיה לו שפע חלב מבהמותיו. ומי שנושאה עליו לא יאונה לו רק טוב. ואם ישימנה בפיו יבלבל דעתו.

33. Galactites: It is somewhat green, and the green is of a somewhat dark shade. And if you look closely—its colour is like ashes of trees. A woman who wants to have much milk should pulverize this stone in whey and drink this [potion] immediately after bathing, before she eats anything else: it tastes like milk, and also looks like it. If someone weaves a thread from the wool of an ewe, perforates this stone, and hangs it around her neck with this thread, she will have plenty of milk. If she [the ewe] has a difficult parturition, he [the shepherd] should attach the stone to her belly, fastened with the mentioned thread.

If someone wants his herd to [produce] much milk, he should wash this stone with pure water and salt and besprinkle his herd with it ere the sun rises: he will then have plenty of milk. No evil will befall him who wears it, but if someone carries it in his mouth, it will confuse his mind. If one holds it against the sun, it will appear full with traversal lines and stripes.

40. GLṬYR' (*galactite*): There are two varieties [of this stone] which can be found in two rivers: the first is the Nile and the second 'YN NYLWS (= Achelous). If a woman wants to have more [breast]milk, she should pulverize [the stone] and drink it immediately after bathing before eating [something]. If someone takes some wool from an ewe, weaves a thread from it, perforates this stone and hangs it around her neck with this thread, she will have plenty of milk. If she [the ewe] has a difficult parturition, he [the shepherd] should attach the stone to her belly, fastened with the same thread as I mentioned.

If someone wants his herd to [produce] much milk, he should pulverize this stone in pure water and salt and besprinkle his herd with the water ere the sun rises: he will then have plenty of milk from his animals. He who wears it, nothing but good will befall him, but if someone carries it in his mouth, it will confuse his mind.

36. דיאַדְקוּדְא. עינה כעין בריל, זכה בכל עבריה. מי שישליך אותה בכלי של מים יוכל לראות כחפצו מ⟨י⟩ן של השדים, והם יענו לו על כל שישאלם, כי אין דבר שיכריח השדים כמוה לדבר כל דבר.על כן קראוה החכמ⟨ים⟩ קדושה, כי מי שיגע עליה מבשר מת או מנבלת עוף ובהמה תאבד כחה.

36. Diadocode: It has the same aspect as beryl, it is pure on all its sides (facets). If someone throws it into a vessel with water, he can see as he pleases a species of demons, and they will answer whatever questions he may ask them. For there is nothing that coerces the demons to speak as well as does [this stone].
The scholars have therefore called it "holy", for if it is brought in contact with a corpse or with the cadaver of a bird or animal, it loses its force.

57. דיאדקודא דומה לאבן בריל ומי שישימנה במים יוכל לראות כחפצו מוצל השדים והם יאמרו לו כל מה שישאל להם.
ומי שיגע
בבשר המת תאבד גבורתה אם אדם בהמה חיה ועוף.

57. DY'DQWD' (*diadocode*). It looks like the beryl. If someone puts it in water, he can see as he pleases the shades of the demons, and they will tell him whatever he asks them.
But if someone touches a corpse with it, or the cadaver of cattle, wild animals or birds, it loses its force.

42. יאייט. קל מאד ושחור לשחרות שבו זך. ומי שיחממו על ידי חיכוך מגביה הקש. ומי שרוצה להבעיר⟨ה⟩ ירחץ האבן במים אז לא יוכל לכבותו כי אם משמן זית.
ומי שחלה מחלי גוטא שהיא בין עור לבשר ישאנו עליו ויגע בו. והמים אשר ירחצוה בהם יחזקו השנים המנענעות. ואם תרצה להשקות אשה ממי רח⟨י⟩צת האבן אם בעולה תשתין מיד ואם לא כן אז היא בתולה בודאי. והעשן מן האבן טוב להזיב נידות. ולשאתה טובה לנכפים ולהבריח שדים. ומי שנהפך בטנו ישתה מגרידת האבן וירפא. ובמים ינתן ג׳ ימים לרפא החלאים שהזכרנו ומי שרייתה יתירו חבלי יולידה. והנפוח ישאנו.

42. Jaiet: It is very light and black. It is of a pure blackness. If someone chafes it by rubbing, it raises [i.e. attracts] the straw. If someone wishes to set it ablaze he should wash the stone in water; it cannot then be quenched, except with olive oil.
If someone fell ill with gout, which is between the skin and the flesh, he should wear [this stone] and touch [the affected spot] with it. The water in which the stone was washed strengthens loose teeth. If you want [to know whether a woman is virgin or not, you should] let her drink from the water in which the stone was washed: if she is no longer a virgin, she will urinate immediately, but if she does not, then she is certainly a virgin. The fumes of the stone are good for [the flux of] menstruating women. Wearing it is beneficial for epileptics and for chasing demons away. If someone suffers from an upset stomach he should drink from [water immixed with] the filings [scrapings] of the stone, and he will be cured. And if it is soaked in water for three days, it [i.e. the water in which it was immersed] cures the illnesses mentioned. Likewise, the water in which it has been soaked eases strong labour pains. The one who has a swelling should wear it.

17. ייאייט. מהם ב׳ מינים ושניהם שחורות. והמבעירו אין יכול לכבותו כי אם בשמן זית.
ולגוטא תרפאהו. ורחצה במים היטב ותשקה לאשה אם בעולה מיד תשתין ולבתולה לא. ויחזק שינים המנענעות. והאשה שלא לזוב בימי ווסתה תעשן מן האבן ותזוב.
וטובה לנכפים ולהבריח השדים.
ומי שנהפך ⟨בטנו⟩ ישתה מן המים וירפא. ולמקשה לילד טובה לשתות מן המים עליה. ונמצאים באינגלילטירא ובארץ ליסא.

17. YY'YYṬ (*jaiet*): There are two varieties [of this stone], and both of them are black. If someone sets it ablaze, he cannot quench it, except with olive oil.
It cures gout.
If one washes the stone thoroughly in water and let a woman drink from it: if she is no longer a virgin, she will urinate immediately, but if she is a virgin, then she is certainly a virgin, she will not [urinate immediately]. It [i.e. the water in which it is washed] strengthens loose teeth. If a woman does not have a flux when she has her period, one should fumigate her [from below], for then she will menstruate. It is beneficial for epileptics and for chasing demons away. If someone suffers from an upset stomach he should drink from its water, for then he will be cured. If a woman has a difficult childbirth, it is good for her to drink from the water [and to put the stone on her belly]. They are found in England and in the land of Lycia.

43. יְרַיְיטא. שחורה קצת. מי שרוחץ פניו תחילה וישים א⟨ו⟩תה בפיו יוכל להבין מה יחשב חבירו עליו. ומה שישאל מן האנשים לא ימנעו ממנ⟨ו⟩. ומן הנשים יעשה חפצו. ומברחת הזב⟨ובים⟩. ובחינת האבן: הנותנה בפיו יטעם טעם דבש. ואפילו אם ימשחו האבן מחלב או מדבש אז יברחו ממנה הזבובים, ובעת יסירו ⟨אותה⟩ ישובו למקומן.

43. Gerachite: It is somewhat black. If someone first washes his face and then puts it in his mouth, he can apprehend what his companion thinks of him. Whatever he may ask of people they will not deny him. With women he can do as he pleases.
It chases flies away. As for testing [the stone]: if one puts it in his mouth, he will perceive a taste like honey. Even if the stone is coated with milk or honey, it will chase the flies. But when the stone is removed they return to where they were.

29. ירייטא. מי שרוחצה במים וישים אותה בפיו יוכל לדעת מה יחשוב עליו חבירו ולא ישיב כל איש פניו ריקם ממה שישאל להם. ומן הנשים יעשה חפצו. ומי שימשח גופו מחלב או מדבש יברחו הדבורים ממנו בהיות זאת האבן עליו ועת יסירנה ממנו ישובו להלחם בו בחזקה.

29. YRYYṬ' (*gerachite*): If someone first washes it in water and then puts it in his mouth, he will be able to know what his companion thinks of him. No one will turn away his request. With women he can do as he pleases. If someone anoints his body with milk or honey, flies will flee from him as long as he wears this stone. But when he removes it they will return to attack him fiercely.

---

44. יֵילַצַא. היא כעין כפור שקורין גרזיל, ולא גדולה ממנו אלא ⟨...⟩. ולעולם היא קרה, ולא בצלולת אש תוכל לחממה. ומי שנושאה בפיו תחת לשונו יבין קצת העתידות. והנושאה לא יירא מאש. והרוצ⟨ה⟩ לדעת עתידות ישימנה בפיו לעת צהרים בחידוש הירח, כי כן כחה. והיא מן מיני גונים מבהיקין למראה העין. ועיגולים סביב לה.

44. Gelazia: It looks like hail which is called *gresil* and is not larger than it, but ⟨...⟩. It is always cold and you cannot heat it [even] by pure fire. Whoever carries it in his mouth under his tongue will know some of the future occurrences. He who wears it need not fear fire. If someone wishes to know future occurrences, he should put it in his mouth at midday at the time of the New Moon, for such is its power. It belongs to the kinds [of stones] whose colours shine when looked at. It has circles around it.

35. יֵילַסְא. כעין כפור שקורין גרישלא היא וקטנה כמוה. ולעולם היא קרה ולא תוכל לחממה כי על יד אש.

35. YeYLaSə' (*gelace*): It looks like hail which is called *gresil* and it is just as small. It is always cold and you cannot heat it, except through fire.

47. מֵידו. רבים ניסו גבורת⟨ה⟩ לאשר עיניו נתעורו על ידי חולי. לקוח זאת האבן וימסכנה בחלב אשה אשר ילדה זכר, וימשח עיניו עד שוב אורו. ולגוטא יושם ⟨ב⟩חלב עז וישתה נסתיקומי [?]. ולכאב חלצים ימשחם מן החלב. והרוצה לעוור אויבו ישחיז האבן במשחזת אדומה במים צלולים וימשח מהן מצח אויבו—מיד ⟨ית⟩עור. ואם תשקהו מן המים יקיא עד שימות. שחורה קראוה מכיר⟨י⟩ה, אבל בתולדתה תמצא ירקרקת. ובעת ירצו לפעול ממנה להטיב: ירקרוקה לבנה; להרע: שחורה.

47.* Medo (*medus*): Many have tried its power for someone whose eyes have been blinded through an illness. One should take this stone, mix it [i.e. its powder] with the milk of a woman who gave birth to a male child, and apply it to his eyes until his eyesight is restored. And for gout one should immerse it in the milk of a goat and let [the patient] drink it [...]. For pain in the loins, one should rub them with the milk.
If someone wants to blind his enemy he should whet the stone on a red whetstone, [immersed] in clear water and rub some of it [i.e. the water with the stone particles] on the forehead of his enemy: he will instantly be blinded. If you let him drink from this water, he will vomit until he dies. The connoisseurs called it "black", but in its nature one also finds a greenish [shade]. When one wants to use [the stone] to do well, [he should employ] the greenish-white one; to do harm, [one should employ] the black one.

34. מידון. זאת האבן נמצאת בארץ מינדא היא מדין. ואיש שהתעוור מחמת חולי יקח זאת האבן וימסכנה בחלב עז אשר ילדה. יועיל לפואקרא. וטוב הוא למי שלא יוכל להוציא נשימתו כי אם בחוזק. אך החלב בכוס כסף וישתה ואליבא ריקנא. ולכאב חלצים ימשח מן החלב. ומי שרוצה לעוור אויבו ישחק מן האבן הזאת במשחזת אדומה במים צלולים וימשח מצח אויבו ויתעוור בשתי עיניו. ואם תשקהו מן המים יקיא עד שימות. ונמצאת ירוקה ובעת שיפעלו ממנה לטובה יקראוה ירוקה ולרעה יקראוה שחורה.

34. MYDWN (*medus*): This stone is found in the land of MYNDʾ which is MDYN (i.e. Media). Someone who has become blind because of an illness should take this stone (i.e. its powder), dilute it with milk of a goat that has given birth. It is beneficial for gout (PWʾQRʾ). It is good for someone who can only breathe with difficulty. One should drink just the milk in a silver cup on an empty stomach. For pain in the loins, one should rub them with the milk. If someone wants to blind his enemy, he should whet the stone on a red whetstone, [immersed] in clear water and rub [some of it] on the forehead of his enemy: he will be blinded in both eyes. If you let him drink from the water, he will vomit until he dies. One can also find a green [variety]. When it is used to do well, it is called "green", and [when it is used] to harm, it is called "black".

49. פַּנְטֵירָא. מן ישפה היא, אבל היא מן גוונים ירוק שחור ואדום. וקצת כהה, אבל זהר יצא מכל גון וגון. הנושאה ויביט עליה טרם זרוח השמש כל איש ירא מפניו, ואותו יום לא ינצח בו במלחמה.	51. פנטירא. מיני גוונים יש בה אדום שחור ירוק והיא כהה אבל זכה בכל מיני גוונים שבה. ואדם שישאנה עליו ויביט בה טרם זרוח ⟨השמש⟩ כל אדם יירא מפניו, ואותו יום שיראנה לא ינוצח במלחמה. ואם נגנב לך שום דבר גע אל הדלת ז׳ פעמים ולא ילך הגנב בשום מקום וחיה יש בארץ אינדא ששמה פנטירא, וכל חיה השומעת קולה תברח מן האריות. והאבן וחיה שוים בכח ובגבורה.
49. Pantera: It is a kind of jasper, but its colors are green, black and red. It is somewhat dark, yet a luminescence issues from each color. If someone wears it and looks at it before sunrise, he will be feared by everyone and will be invincible in battle on that day.	51. PNṬYR' (*pantera*): It has different colors [like] red, black and green. It is dark but pure in all its different colors. If someone wears it and looks at it before sunrise, he will be feared by everyone and will be invincible on the day that he looks at it. In case something has been stolen from you, touch the door seven times [with this stone] and the thief will not go anywhere. There is an animal in the land of India called "panther". Every [other] animal, [even lions], that hears its voice flees for it. The stone and the animal [i.e. panther] are equal in power and force.
60. קַלְקוּפִינָא. שחורת על פני כולה. ואם תכה עליה בפטיש ישמע כקול למרחוק, כמו מכה על מחבת נחשת. הנושאה בלא טינוף שגל יהיה לו לעולם קול ערב.	53. קלקופיינא. שחורה היא כולה ואם תכה עליה תשמע קולה כמו מחבת. ומי שנושאה עליו בלא משכבי אשה לעולם יהיה קולו ערב.
60. *Calcofine (*calcofone*): It is black in its entirety. If you strike it with a hammer a sound will be heard far away, like when one strikes a bronze frying pan. The one who wears it without being defiled through cohabitation will always have a pleasant voice.	53. QLQWPYYN' (*calcofone*): It is completely black. If you strike it, you will hear a sound like [when one strikes] a frying pan. The one who wears it without being defiled through cohabitation will always have a pleasant voice.

56. קוֹרְטוֹלִינַא. אדומה כולה והאדום אופל מאד ועיקר מראית⟨ה⟩ כמים שרחצו בו בשר. הנושאה באצבעו או בצוארו יהיה קשה לכעוס ונוח לרצות. מעמדת הדם בכל מקום שהוא, אחר אשר יבש הדם עליה מחום השמש או מחם האש. ולעצור זיבת האשה טוב מאד.	21. קרנוליאה. אדומה כולה והאודם אפל מאד ודומה למים אשר רוחץ בה בשר. והנושאה באצבעו או בצוארו יהיה קשה לכעוס ונוח לרצות. ומעמדת הדם בכל מקום שהוא עליה. גם לזיבת ⟨האישה⟩ טובה מאד.
56. *Cortolina (*cornoligne*): It is thoroughly red, and the red is very dark: it basically looks like water that has been used to wash meat. Whoever wears it on his finger or his neck will be little irascible and easy to appease. It stops bleeding anywhere [in the body], [namely,] after the blood on it has dried through the heat of the sun or the heat of fire. It is very beneficial to stop [excessive] menstrual bleeding of a woman.	21. QRNWLY'H (*cornoligne*): It is completely red, and the red is very dark: it looks like water that has been used to wash meat. Whoever wears it on his finger or his neck will be little irascible and easy to appease. It stops bleeding anywhere [in the body], [namely,] after the blood on it has dried. It is very beneficial to stop [excessive] menstrual bleeding of a woman.

SUPPLEMENT B

THE *KO'AḤ HA-AVANIM* IN ITS FRENCH CONTEXT: ROMANCE AND LATIN TERMS AND SOURCES

1. *Introduction*[*]

Berakhyah Ben Natronai ha-Nakdan's lapidary *Ko'aḥ ha-Avanim* contains a certain number of Old French—more precisely Anglo-Norman—and Latin words, written in Hebrew characters. In contrast to the Hebrew text, these elements are mostly vocalized with a punctuation system that follows by and large the Tiberian tradition. The use of the vernacular language and Latin concerns the names of the 72 stones—with the exception of stones no. 68–70 that have Hebrew names—as well as over 30 terms within the Hebrew continuous text. These terms refer, inter alia, to other stones, diseases and plants.[1]

The use of Hebrew characters for non-Hebrew purposes was not unusual. In the Old Testament already, Aramaic passages have been written in Hebrew characters,[2] and especially from the Middle Ages, many Hebrew written texts in several languages have been passed down to us. Numerous Judeo-Arabic texts are known, particularly from Muslim ruled Spain, where Moses Maimonides (1138–1204), e.g., wrote almost all his works in Arabic.[3] Other languages of the Jewish diaspora, for instance Greek,[4] Persian[5] and Romance languages like Spanish,[6] Catalan,

* I sincerely thank Guido Mensching for his useful comments to an earlier version of this introduction.

1 Cf. section 2.

2 Cf. Kramer & Kowallik (1994:XII).

3 Cf. Halkin (1971:410); Rabinowitz (1971:754).

4 Cf. Dalven (1971:425 ff.).

5 Cf. Fischel (1971:429 ff.).

6 Cf. Kramer & Kowallik (1994:XIV). In contrast to the other mentioned languages, Judeo-Spanish has a special status, since here we have an idiom of archaic Spanish, spoken by the Jewish who were expelled from Spain at the end of the 16th c. and who settled down particularly in the region of the former Ottoman Empire. Judeo-Spanish is known in two variants—the vernacular so called *djudezmo* and the literary *ladino*—and differs linguistically from the standard Spanish spoken on the peninsula (cf. Sala 1998:375).

Occitan,[7] Italian[8] and French were also put down by means of the Hebrew alphabet.[9] Whereas Judeo-Spanish documents are extant in large numbers, French texts in Hebrew characters are more rarely known. Famous examples are Rashi's glosses in his commentary on the Talmud (11th c., translations of difficult Aramaic and Hebrew words into the *la'az*),[10] the poetic work *Poèmes judéo-français du Moyen Age*,[11] and the 13th c.'s medical compilation *Fevres* treating the causes, symptoms and therapy of fevers.[12] In contrast to the last two mentioned continuous texts, the *Ko'aḥ ha-Avanim* has only single detached Romance and Latin words within the Hebrew text (cf. above).

1.1. *The Language*

The language of these non-Hebrew words (stone names and other terms) can definitely be identified as partly a dialect of O. Fr., namely Angl.-Nor., and partly as Lat. In the case of Romance words, the O. Fr. terms correspond in large part both to the Francien[13] and the Angl.-Nor.[14] dialect. This is due, on the one hand, to the fact that the medieval mineralogical terminology consists almost throughout of scientific Gr.-Lat. loan-words, which were not submitted to all the specific sound shifts of the dialects. On the other hand, regional written dialects began since the second half of the 12th c. to be orientated towards the Francien dialect, the surroundings of Paris being the politically and economically dominating region.[15]

---

[7] Occitan and Catalan words written in Hebrew characters can be found and are analysed, e.g., in Bos/ Mensching et al. (edition of the 29th book of the *Sefer ha-Shimmush*, a Hebrew-Arabic-Romance synonym list; forthcoming); Bos & Mensching (2005); Mensching & Savelsberg (2004); Bos & Mensching (2001).

[8] Cf. Sala (1998:384ff.).

[9] Cf. Kramer (1996:591ff.).

[10] Ed. Darmesteter & Blondheim (1929).

[11] Ed. Blondheim (1927).

[12] This comprehensive anonymous treatise (almost 400 folios filled recto and verso) is the purpose of several editions (cf. Oesterreicher 1896; Katzenellenbogen 1933; Kiwitt 2001) and actual edition projects (cf. Zaun 2002; Zwink 2006; Zwink unedited).

[13] Francien was the prevailing O. Fr. dialect, spoken in the region Ile-de-France, which forms the basis of standard Mod. Fr.; the common O. Fr. dictionaries list the headwords in Francien.

[14] Angl.-Nor. is a dialect of the *langue d'oïl*, which was brought into England by the Norman upper class following the Norman conquest in 1066 and which differed phonologically and lexicologically from the dialect of the Ile-de-France.

[15] Cf. Vossler (1929:15).

The Romance terms in the *Ko'aḥ ha-Avanim* can clearly be identified as O. Fr. or Angl.-Nor. The ending of words in [ə] < Lat. -A (Hebrew transcription with final alef, often vocalized with sheva) excludes other Romance languages like Spanish, Catalan, Occitan, Portuguese, and Italian, which would show for the corresponding words the conservation of final [a], e.g.,

(1) entry no. 48: פֵּירְלְא (*PeYRLə'*) is O. Fr. / Angl.-Nor. *perle*, 'pearl' (TL 7:762; FEW 8:253b; AND 5:518b); by contrast, we have in O. Sp. *perla* (DETEMA 2:1209a), O. Cat. id. (DCVB 8:478b), O. Occ. id. (FEW 8:253b), O. Port. *pérola* (DHLP 2191c), O. It. *pirla* (GDLI 13:50b), stemming all from Lat. PERNA (see FEW 8:253a).

Another clear indication of Fr. is the presence of some terms that are hereditarily existant only in the *langue d'oïl*, e.g.,

(2) entry no. 39: גֵייטְא (*GeYYṬ'ə*) and entry no. 42: יאייט (*Y'YYṬ*) represent O. Fr. *jaiet* / Angl.-Nor. *gaiet* / *gagate*, 'jet' (TL 4:1544; FEW 4:21a; AND 3:325b); O. Sp. has *azavache* (Sin. 114, fn. 19), O. Cat. *atzabeja* (DCVB 2:136b);[16]

(3) entry no. 44: גרזיל (*GRZYL*) is O. Fr. / Angl.-Nor. *gresil(le)*, 'hail' (TL 4:626; FEW 16:85b–86a; AND 3:342a), a term of Frankish origin; by contrast, we find in O. Sp. *granizo* (DETEMA 1:786b); Cat. *calamarsa* (DCVB 2:834a); O. Occ. *peyra* or *granha* (DAO 117); It. *grandine* (REW 3843).

Since Berakhyah lived and worked in Normandy,[17] it stands to reason to examine the language in view of the Angl.-Nor. dialect. As a result, it can be said that almost all Romance terms that were identified as O. Fr. can also be interpreted as Angl.-Nor. In some cases, terms appear even in variants that are only attested for Angl.-Nor., e.g.,

(4) entry no. 38: אֲצִיר (*'aZiYR*) is Angl.-Nor. *ascir*, 'steel' (documented only in the online version of the AND);[18] for Francien, indeed, only diphthongized forms like *acier* (TL 1:86b; FEW 24:104b) are attested;

(5) entry no. 39: וינש (*WYNŠ*) is the plural of Angl.-Nor. *vene*, 'vein' (AND 7:849b); by contrast, in Francien, we find only diphthongized forms like *veine* (TL 11:139; FEW 14:226a).

16 O. Occ. *jaiet* and It. *giaietto* are borrowings from O. Fr. (cf. FEW 4:21b).
17 Cf. Introduction to the text edition.
18 See URL: http://www.anglo-norman.net/gate/ s.v. *acer* (31st oct. 2007).

Moreover, we deal in the *Ko'aḥ ha-Avanim* with words that are exclusively documented for Angl.-Nor., e.g.,

(6) entry no. 46: דֵיטְא (*DeYṬə'*) for *date*, 'urine' (AND 2:140b; FEW 21:318b);

(7) entry no. 50: פִּידוֹרַטַשׁ (*PiYDWoRaṬaŠ*) for Angl.-Nor. *pedoretes*, 'paederos, a stone' (AND 5:509b = CL 1367);

(8) entry no. 63: שׁוֹלְנִיטֵי (*ŠWLNiYṬeY*) for *solenite*, 'selenite, moonstone' (AND 6:711).

From the total 84 non-Hebrew stone names, 60 were identified as O. Fr. and/or Angl.-Nor. (approximately 71 %). The remaining 21 terms are Lat. (25 %),[19] which are, like the following examples no. (9)–(11) show, often variants that are only attested in Mediaeval Latin texts. The mineralogical terminology goes either back to Gr. (in most cases), e.g.,

(9) entry no. 31: גרישופציאון (*GRYŠWPṢY'WN*) is M. Lat. *crisopacion* (variant of Lat. *chrysoprasus*[20] < Gr. χρυσόπρασος), 'species gemmae (chrysoprase)' (MLWB 2:561);

(10) entry no. 71: צִילִידוֹנְיָא (*ṢiYLiYDoWNəYa'*) is *cilidonia*, a M. Lat. variant of Lat. *chelidonia* (< Gr. χελιδόνιος), 'chelidony' (MLWB 2:531; ThLL 3:1004),

or is borrowed from Arab., e.g.,[21]

(11) entry no. 25: אַנְשְׂרָא (*'aNŠRa'*) for M. Lat. *ambra* (< Arab. *'anbar*) 'excrementa piscis, ambergis' (MLWB 1:549).

Regarding the non-Hebrew linguistic material at large (i.e., including the terms featuring within the Hebrew text), we can say that almost all 103 terms could be identified concerning their language and meaning. The linguistic distribution of these terms is as follows: approximately 80 % of the lexies are Romance, 20 % are Lat. From the Romance terms, 82 % are both documented for generally O. Fr. and Angl.-Nor., whereas 12 % feature only in Angl.-Nor. texts; 7 % of the Romance words are not especially attested for Angl.-Nor., but for other O. Fr. dialects (e.g., Francien). One word is a transcription of Greek; cf. the following table:

---

[19] The language of 3 stone names could not be identified.

[20] Featuring, e.g., in Pliny nat. XXXVII, 77.

[21] Generally, 80 % of the Lat. mineralogical nomenclature is of Gr. origin; only a few "pure" Lat. exist (cf. Goltz 1972:381–382).

Language	All non-Hebrew terms	Stone names
Latin	22	21
O. Fr. / Angl.-Nor.	64	55
Only Angl.-Nor.	10	4
Other O. Fr. dialect or other language	6	4
Greek	1	–
Total amount	103	84

The high rate of Romance lexemes in a scientific text may astonish, since the vernacular has mostly been considered as the language of the regional and common registers, whereas the scientific language of the Middle Ages was, according to the common perception, Lat.[22] However, this opinion can be confuted by many editors of Judeo-Romance texts: Kiwitt showed in his edition of the cited Judeo-Fr. medical treatise *Fevres* that O. Fr. as a scientific language was much more developed than it was supposed to be;[23] the same observation was made, also for O. Fr., by the author[24] and, for O. Occ. / O. Cat., by Bos and Mensching.[25] Secondly, it must be said that the vernacular terms are rarely hereditary words and in large part scientific Gr.-Lat. loan-words (cf. above), which have certainly penetrated the O. Fr. / Angl.-Nor. vocabulary, but often only with an adapted ending, e.g.,

(12) entry no. 28: בֵּירֵיל (*BeYReYL*), O. Fr. / Angl.-Nor. *beril*, 'beryl', is adopted from Gr.-Lat. BERYLLUS (TL 1:928; FEW 1:339b; AND 1:67a).

Before we get onto a closer look on specific linguistic problems concerning Romance words in Hebrew transcription, we would like to stress at the outset that we do not deal with Judeo-Fr. in the sense of a special language that has its origins in the Lat. of the Bible and that was only spoken by the Jewish population of France. This hypothesis of a Jewish Fr. language, different from the Fr. spoken by the non-Jewish population, was made by Blondheim[26] and later on corroborated by, e.g., Levy, Weinreich and Wexler.[27] The opposite opinion has always been advanced

[22] Cf. Müller (1975:148).
[23] Cf. Kiwitt (2001:41).
[24] Cf. Zwink (2006:253); Zwink (unedited).
[25] Cf. Mensching & Savelsberg (2004); Bos & Mensching (2005); Bos/ Mensching et al. (forthcoming).
[26] Cf. Blondheim (1925).
[27] Cf. Levy (1932) and (1964); Weinreich (1956); Wexler (1981). The FEW also denotes certain variants with the label "jud. fr.", i.e., 'Judeo-Fr.'.

by Romance philologists;[28] the most detailed and convincing argumentation against a specific Judeo-Fr. language can be found in Banitt's article "Une langue fantôme: le judéo-français", where he reasoned: "Abandonnons [...] toute idée préconçue d'un parler particulier aux Juifs de France", and below, "il n'y a [...] pas de pénétration hétérogène, ni dans le système phonétique, ni dans le système morphologique. [...] Abordons [...] les documents en question comme toute autre document ancien français."[29] Banitt's observation can be confirmed against the backdrop of our research results: the Romance linguistic material of the *Ko'aḥ ha-Avanim* is conform with the variants given in the standard dictionaries of O. Fr. and Angl.-Nor.[30]

1.2. *Lexicological and Graphical Problems*

However, Romance texts in Hebrew transcription present a specific set of difficulties regarding to two main aspects, with which we are also faced in the *Ko'aḥ ha-Avanim*. The first aspect refers to lexicological problems, the second to the way of representing non-Hebrew words by Hebrew characters.

1.2.1. Lexicological Aspects

The lexicological problems of the Romance/ Latin elements to which we are confronted in Berakhyahs lapidary can be subsumed under two main categories: first, a lacking documentation of the term for the relevant epoch (Middle Ages), and secondly, no documentation at all, so that the meaning of the term remains unclear. These divergencies from attested lexemes provide new informations about the Fr. mineralogical terminology in the Middle Ages; cf. the following exemples.[31]

The first mentioned lexicological problem, i.e., the documentation of some lexemes in the standard dictionaries of O. Fr. and Angl.-Nor.[32]

[28] Cf. Sala (1998:373).
[29] Banitt (1963:292).
[30] Cf. section 2.
[31] For a detailed discussion of the single terms, cf. section 2.
[32] The systematically consulted dictionaries are, for O. Fr., the TL (= Tobler & Lommatzsch 1925–1976, *Altfranzösisches Wörterbuch*) and the FEW (= *Französisches Etymologisches Wörterbuch*, ed. by von Wartburg, 1922–); for Angl.-Nor., the FEW and the AND (= *Anglo-Norman Dictionary*, ed. by Stone & Rothwell, 1977–1992).

for only later language epochs should be illustrated by the following exemples. For these words, we might assume a very first documentation in the *Ko'aḥ ha-Avanim*:

> (13) entry no. 17: אִירְוֹנְא (*'iYRWoNə'*) / אירונא (*'YRWN'*) must designate a kind of stone—and not O. Fr. / Angl.-Nor. *irai(g)ne*, 'spider', see TL 4:1433; FEW 25–1:77b–78a; AND 3:364b). However, the FEW (25–1:80b) gives another derivation from Lat. ARANEA, namely the Mod. Fr. (18th c.) *arannea* referring to a "minerai d'argent composé de fils d'argent" (i.e., silver mineral, built out of silver fibres). We might thus probably assume that something like *iraine* / **irone* also designated a kind of stone or mineral, and this already in the 12th/13th c.;
>
> (14) entry no. 27: אַמַאוּנְטְשׁ (*'aMa'uWNṬŠ)* might refer to Fr. *amiantes*, plural of *amiante*, 'kind of asbestos', which is, according to the FEW (24:437a), only documented for M. and Mod. Fr. If we really deal with a Romance form here (and not with the Lat. *amiantus*, cf. ThLL 1:1889), the *Ko'aḥ ha-Avanim* would give us here a first documentation of this Fr. form.

Another difficulty consists in word compositions, whose single components are well documented in the dictionaries; the compound term, however, is missing in the sources and features only in the present edition, so that we can assume here also a first documentation, e.g.,

> (15) entry no. 62: שפיר אורי׳אנט (*ŠPYR 'WRY'NṬ)* consists of the O. Fr. / Angl.-Nor. elements *saphir*, 'sapphire' (TL 9:39: FEW 12:213a; AND 6:667a) and *orient*, 'east, orient' (TL 6:1270: FEW 7:413a; AND 4:469b), thus **saphir orient*, and means literally 'sapphire of the orient, oriental sapphire'; the combination of these two elements is not attested in the consulted sources;
>
> (16) entry no. 62: יגונצא מרינא (*YGWNṢ' MRYN'*), **jagonce marine*, is the combination of the O. Fr. / Angl.-Nor. elements *jagonce*, 'jacinth' (TL 4:1537; FEW loc. cit.; AND 3:367b) and *marine*, 'marine' (TL 5:1173; FEW 6–1:344b; AND 4:407b) and has the literal meaning 'marine, watery jacinth'; the compound term is not documented in the sources.

In some cases, the Ms. shows forms that are not documented for Romance languages, but for which we must assume a (spontaneous?) creation of a O. Fr / Angl.-Nor. variant modelled upon a Lat. basis, e.g.,

> (17) entry no. 45: לְיְנֶיטְא (*LəYNeYṬə'*) seems to represent a non-documented O. Fr. / Angl.-Nor. loan-word **legnete*, formed upon the Lat. *lignita*, 'lychnis; a stone' (ThLL 7:1939). The ending in [ə] of our variant suggests a O. Fr. / Angl.-Nor. and not a Lat. reading.

The second main lexicological problem we would like to mention is the presence of some lexies that could not be identified at all, concerning both form and meaning, e.g.,

(18) entry no. 51: פַּיְיטוֹרוֹשׁ (*PaYəYṬoWRWoŠ*) suggests something like **paietoros*. The identity of this term (designating a stone) is unclear;

(19) entry no. 62: the form עלישטרא (*'LYŠTR̤'*), **alestre* or the like, must also remain unexplained.

1.2.2. Graphical Aspects

Concerning the Hebrew transcription of Romance and Lat. words in the *Ko'aḥ ha-Avanim*, we are confronted with difficulties that all these texts have in common: phonemes must be transcribed that do not have equivalents in Hebrew and for which the scribe can thus be less oriented towards a tradition of graphical representation. Since the present edition of the *Ko'aḥ ha-Avanim* is not based on an autograph manuscript but on a 14th c. copy, we have to consider not only O. Fr. and Angl-.Nor. phonological particularities of the composition epoch (probably the beginning of the 13th c.), but also have to include sound changes that took place until the date of the creation of the Ms. copy. In the following, only a few selected problems are mentioned:[33]

A prevalent problem concerns the representation of the vowels [i] and [e]. The confusion of these vowels is typical for Fr. texts in Hebrew transcription and is possibly due to the proximity of their articulation: both sounds are palatal vowels and are adjacent concerning the height ([i] is a close, [e] a mid vowel). This oscillation can also be found in the cited medical treatise *Fevres*, cf., e.g., נִינוֹפַר (*NiYNWoPaR*) for *nenufar*, 'water lily' (fol. 158b–8), or שֵׁינוֹכָא (*ŠeYNWoKa'*) for *sinocha*, 'synocha, a kind of fever' (fol. 163b–8).[34] In the *Ko'aḥ ha-Avanim*, this phenomenon appears quite often, e.g.

(20) entry no. 6: אִיטִיטְא (*'iYṬiṬə'*) representing O. Fr. / Angl.-Nor. *et(h)ite*, 'aetites, eagle-stone' (TL 3:1519; FEW 24:240a; AND 2:285a) shows a vocalization of the first syllable with ḥireq, whereas only variants with initial [e] are documented in our sources;

(21) entry no. 12: אוֹרֵיטא (*'WoReYṬ'*), O. Fr. or Angl.-Nor. *orit(h)e*, 'a precoius stone, oritis' (TL 6:1285; FEW 7:417a; AND 4:469b), represents

[33] In section 2, graphical and phonological problems are discussed for every single O. Fr. / Angl.-Nor. term.

[34] Cf. Zwink (unedited).

the inverse case, i.e., the resh is punctuated with a tsere, which should, indeed, be pronounced [ri].

Another frequent oscillation of vowelization concerns the the sounds [a] and [e], which are also two adjacent vowles with respect to their articulation (open and mid vowel, respectively). We sometimes find a Hebrew punctuation with tsere, actually representing [e], where we would expect a patach representing [a]. The inverse case, i.e., patach instead of tsere, occurs just as often; cf. the following exemples:

(22) entry no. 14: אֵימַטִישְׁא (*'eYMaṬiYŠə'*), O. Fr. / Angl.-Nor. *ametiste*, 'amethyst' (TL 1:349; FEW 24:436a; AND 1:25b), shows a vowelization with tsere of initial alef and with patach in the second syllable, which would suggest a non-documented variant like **ematice*. Since the same phenomenon appears in quite frequent other cases, we might rather suppose a particularity of this text than erroneous transcriptions.

(23) entry no. 33: גַלַקְטִיטַשׁ (*GaLaQṬiYṬaŠ*) is Lat. *galactites*, 'galactite, a stone' (ThLL 6–2:1669). As we can see here, the oscillation between [a] and [e] (here patach instead of tsere in the last syllyble) appears also in Lat. words.

In Angl.-Nor., the sound of final postconsonantal shwa "began to become unstable in the thirteenth century and was more and more frequently effaced."[35] This phonological phenomenon becomes visible in the Hebrew transcription of Angl.-Nor. words in the *Ko'aḥ ha-Avanim*, where final [ə] is sometimes represented by sheva with alef as *mater lectionis* like in

(24) entry no. 48: פֵּירְלְא (*PeYRLə'*), i.e., O. Fr. / Angl.-Nor. *perle*, 'pearl' (TL 7:762; FEW 8:253b; AND 5:518b),

but quite often, the representation of final [ə] is lacking, like, e.g., in

(25) entry no. 10: אַבֵּישְׁט (*'aBeYŠṬ*) for O. Fr. / Angl.-Nor. *abeste*, 'asbestos' (TL 1:559; FEW 25–1:407a; AND 1:2b).

The final graphical particularity concerning vowels we like to mention is the lack of nun or mem indicating the nasalization of preceding vowels. This absence may be interpreted as the representation of weakness or even loss of nasalization which occurs in Late Angl.-Nor.;[36] cf., e.g.,

[35] Pope (1934:438).
[36] Cf. Pope (1934:441–442).

(26) entry no. 53: קַרְבּוֹקְלא (*QaRBoWQL'*) for O. Fr. / Angl.-Nor. *charbo(u)cle / c(h)arbuncle / c(h)arboncle*, 'carbuncle, ruby' (TL 2:256; FEW 2-1:360a; AND 1:91a).

Regarding the graphical representation of consonants, the existence of certain affricate (like /ʧ/ and /ʤ/) and fricative consonants (like /ʒ/), (O.) Fr. peculiarities not known in Hebrew, presents a difficulty for the scribe. The sound shift of the affricate consonants ([ʦ], [ʧ] and [ʤ]) into fricative consonants ([s], [ʃ] and [ʒ]) took place in O. Fr. around 1200,[37] and somewhat later in Angl.-Nor.[38] Since the composition of the *Ko'aḥ ha-Avanim* falls exactly in this transitional period (cf. above), we can not definitely say which sound should be represented. However, the fact that the copy of the Ms. was made in the 14th c. supports the assumption that our text transcribes rather fricative than affricate consonants. So, [ʒ] is represented either by gimmel or by yod, cf. the following examples:

(27) entry no. 39: גֵייטְא (*GeYYṬ'ə*), with initial gimmel, is O. Fr. *jaiet* or Angl.-Nor. *gaiet / gagate*, 'jet' (TL 4:1544; FEW 4:21a; AND 3:325b);

(28) entry no. 42: יאייט (*Y'YYṬ*), with initial yod, represents the same word.

The representation of [ʒ] by yod occurs also in two other cases: יַרַיִיטא (*YaRaYiYṬ'*) for O. Fr. / Angl.-Nor. *gerachite*, 'hieracitis' (see entry no. 43) and יִילַצַא (*YiYLaZa'*) for Lat. *gelazia*, 'hailstone' (see entry no. 44). This way of transcribing [ʒ] can also be found in the cited O. Fr. text *Fevres*,[39] but seems to be absent from Old Occitan (spoken in medieval Southern France) texts in the Sephardic tradition, e.g. the *Sefer ha-Shimmush*[40] or in the *Sharshot ha-Kesef*.[41]

Another problem is the transcription of the O. Fr. palatal consonants [ʎ] and [ɲ]. For Angl.-Nor., we have to note the loss of the palatalization (ordinarily resolved into dental [l] and [n]) of these sounds in the course of the 13th c.,[42] but the pronunciation seemed to vary for some time,[43] and Lat. alphabet based texts show even in the aftermath of the sound shift orthographic variants[44] that indicate that the writers were aware of the

---

[37] Cf. Rheinfelder (1963:164).

[38] Cf. Pope (1934:450).

[39] See Kiwitt (2001:33), who concludes from this way of transcription the loss of affricate consonants; Banitt indeed remarks: "Old French [ʤ] was transcribed by י with a diacritical mark until the 13th century" (Banitt 1971:424).

[40] Ed. Bos/ Mensching et al. (fothcoming).

[41] Ed. Aslanov (2001).

[42] Cf. Menger (1904:88).

[43] Cf. Pope (loc. cit.).

[44] Orthographic variants are documented by Menger (loc. cit.).

former pronunciation. At the time of the composition of the lapidary, the consonants were probably still pronounced in the palatal manner. However, it has to be stressed that the consonants [ʎ] and [ɲ] are—just like in *Fevres*—[45] not labelled by any diacritical mark, but they appear virtually always together with a yod in their phonological environment (following or preceeding), e.g.:

(29) entry no. 19: אופטליאש (*ʾWPṬLYʾŠ*), O. Fr. / Angl.-Nor. *optallie* 'opal' (TL 6:1159; FEW 7:358b; AND 4:466a), has a single lamed, followed by yod;

(30) entry no. 63: מילפוייל (*MYLPWYYL*), O. Fr. / Angl.-Nor. *milfoil*, 'yarrow' (TL 6:47; FEW 6-2:92b; AND 4:427a); final [ʎ] is probably marked by a preceding yod;

(31) entry no. 45: לְינֵיטְא (*LəYNeYṬəʾ*), O. Fr. *legnete for 'lychnis', features with a nun preceded by yod.

Taken as a whole, the above presented specific characteristics of this O. Fr./Angl.-Nor. text in Hebrew transcription show to us some striking details concerning the pronounciation of O. Fr./Angl.-Nor. at this epoch. Firstly, regarding the transcription of the vowels [e] and [i], that is to say the hesitation between these two sounds, we may conclude that the degree of aperture of the mouth (close and close-mid) varied little. The graphical representation shows furthermore that the sound shift from affricate into fricative consonants, which took generally place in O. Fr. around the year 1200, had probably already been concluded at this epoch of Angl.-Nor., as well as the loss of nasalization and the pronunciation of final shwa. Finally, the fact that lamed and nun appear nearly always together with yod when they should be pronounced [ʎ] and [ɲ], might indicate that the sound shift into dental consonants had not been completed.

1.3. *Conventions of Transliteration*

The Hebrew consonants and signs of vowelization are transliterated into a Lat. alphabet based graphical code. For the reader who is less familiar with Hebrew characters, this transliteration aims to facilitate the retracement of the word reconstructions. The conventions follow the ones that were established for the edition of the 29th book of the *Sefer ha-Shimmush*;[46] the principle is to assign to every Hebrew character and

45 Cf. Kiwitt (2001:21); Zwink (2006:257).
46 Ed. Bos/ Mensching et al. (forthcoming), cf. above.

sign of vocalization a Lat. equivalent. Concretely, Hebrew consonants are rendered by Lat. majuscules, and the diacritical vowel signs by Lat. minuscules. An exception concerns the sheva, which is only transcribed if it appears with a *mater lectionis*, i.e., a supporting consonant (mostly alef or yod). In detail, the present edition is based on the following transliteration system:

Consonants

א (alef)	ʾ	ח (ḥet)	Ḥ	ם (mem sofit)	M	צ (tsadi)	Ṣ
ב (bet)	B	ט (ṭet)	Ṭ	נ (nun)	N	ץ (tsadi sofit)	Ṣ
ג (gimmel)	G	י (yod)	Y	ן (nun sofit)	N	ק (qof)	Q
ד (dalet)	D	כ (kaf)	K	ס (samek)	S	ר (resh)	R
ה (he)	H	ך (kaf sofit)	K	ע (ayin)	ʿ	ש (shin)	Š
ו (vav)	W	ל (lamed)	L	פ (pe)	P	ת (tav)	T
ז (zayin)	Z	מ (mem)	M	ף (pe sofit)	P		

Vowel signs[47]

◌ַ (patach)	a	◌ֵ (tsere)	e	◌ֹ (ḥolem)	o	◌ְ (sheva)	ə
◌ָ (qamets)	a	◌ִ (ḥireq)	i	◌ֻ (qibbuts)	u		

1.4. *The Sources*

Berakhyah used mainly Angl.-Nor. mineralogical compilations as source and model both for the selection and for the description of the virtues of the stones.[48] Altogether, 15 Angl.-Nor. and Lat. texts were identified as possible sources, whereas it turned out in the course of our study that the Cambridge Lapidary (CL), a Angl.-Nor. Marbode translation,[49] must have been used as main source text for Berakhyah.[50] Firstly, the *Ko'aḥ ha-Avanim* shows conspicuously often very close parallels to this text, and in many cases, we have even the impression of literal translations.[51] Secondly, some stones discussed by Berakhyah feature exclusively in the CL, so that we have to assume a direct relation between Berakhyah

[47] Only vowels signs featuring in the text are presented and transliterated here.

[48] For an overview over the history of the lapidary tradition, cf. the introduction to the text edition.

[49] Ed. Studer & Evans (1924). This version was made directly from the Lat. text and is not dependent, like the other Angl.-Nor. versions, on the First French Version (cf. Studer & Evans 1924:154).

[50] In section 3, the information which Berakhyah gives for the single stones is traced back to its assumed sources.

[51] Cf., among many others, stones no. 4 (*esmeralde*), 7 (*eliotrope*), 18 (*androdragme*), 32 (*gagatrome*).

and this text.[52] And finally, the graphical representation of the *Ko'aḥ ha-Avanim* corresponds often to the spelling of the CL; cf., e.g., stone no. 20, where our אַבְשִׁיטַא (*'aBŠiYṬa'*) corresponds to the Angl.-Nor. variant *absite* featuring in CL 1245 (in contrast to O. Fr. *absicte*).

In much less frequent cases, other Angl.-Nor. Marbode translations show closer parallels than the CL.[53] Sometimes, we could also identify Lat. texts—here mostly the 16th book of Isidore's *Etymologiae*—as a source.[54] These cases are rare, and we must probably assume that an intermediate text, unknown to us, was at Berakhyah's disposal. Moreover, Berakhyah must have had access to at least one more text that we do not know at all, which was supposably Hebrew. The traditions about stones no. 68–70 may go back to this source, since, firstly, the designations of these stones are in Hebrew and, secondly, the mentioned traditions could not be traced back to a source text that is known to us. The fact that sometimes for single traditions[55] or even for the whole stone description[56] given by Berakhyah no parallels could be retrieved, may also indicate that another text must have existed, which was used a as source by Berakhyah.

1.5. *Structure of* Supplement B

This present *Supplement B* contains the following sections: in section 2, we present a detailed lexicological commentary on the Romance and Lat. terminology; section 3 contains a systematic analysis of Berakhyah's sources with respect to the different traditions listed by him regarding the provenance, physical aspect, supposed virtues of the stones; section 4 contains tables of sources. Afterwards, three glossaries are added with the objective of facilitating the consultation of the Romance and Lat. terms. The first glossary is arranged according to the Hebrew transcription and gives the corresponding Romance or Lat. designation, followed by a reference to the stone number assigned in the edition. The second and third glossary present the inverse case: they are arranged according to the Romance / Lat. or Greek designation, respectively, and refer to

[52] Cf., e.g., stones no. 13 (*enidre*) and 50 (*pedoretes*).

[53] E.g., the First French Version and the Alphabetical Lapidary for stone no. 2 (*acates*).

[54] E.g., stones no. 22 (*optallius*) and 26 (*astrites*).

[55] Cf., among many others, stones no. 2 (*acates*), 9 (*ematis*), 28 (*beril*), 29 (*grisoloite*).

[56] Cf., e.g., stones no. 24 (**asyctus*), 25 (*ambra*), 27 (*amiantus*), 51 (*paederos*), 52 (**peritora*).

the Hebrew transcription as well as to the number of the stone in the edition. *Supplement B* is concluded by a bibliography containing works which are cited in particular in this present supplement B.

2. *Lexicological Commentary on the Romance and Latin Terms*

This commentary on the single O. Fr. / Angl.-Nor. and Lat. lexemes in the *Koʾaḥ ha-Avanim* is structured in the following way: The stone names feature in the same order as they appear in the Ms. and are numbered consecutively in accordance with the text edition. The glossaries also refer to those numbers.

In the first line of a commentary, the Hebrew term (bold) is quoted, followed by its transliteration (italic; for the conventions of transliteration, cf. section 1). In the next line, the term is discussed with respect to its language (in the majority of cases O. Fr. / Angl.-Nor. or Lat.), the attested variants that might be represented by the Hebrew term, and its meaning as given in the dictionaries. The references of the documenting sources feature then in parentheses (for the abbreviations, cf. the bibliography). Our main sources are, for the Romance languages, the most comprehensive standard lexicon of O. Fr., i.e., the Tobler-Lommatzsch (TL), the etymological lexicon of Walter von Wartburg (FEW), and the *Anglo-Norman Dictionary* (AND, ed. Rothwell), which incorporates the Angl.-Nor. Marbode translations (cf. section 4 of the introduction to the edition). For the Lat. terms, the *Mittellateinisches Wörterbuch* (MLWB, available until *ev-*), the *Thesaurus Linguae Latinae* (ThLL, available until *p-*), and, for the terms beginning with characters following later in the alphabet, the *Lateinisch-deutsches Handwörterbuch* (GH, ed. Georges) or the *Lexicon Totius Latinitatis* (LTL, ed. Forcellini) was used. If a word is not documented in the mentioned dictionaries, primary text sources were consulted additionally (for the abbreviations, cf. the bibliography).

Particularities and difficulties concerning the meaning, the language, the (first) documentation, and the Hebrew graphical representation of the Romance or Lat. word (e.g., erroneous or unclear transcription) are discussed subsequently.

Romance and Lat. words featuring in the continuous Hebrew text are treated in same way as described above and are commented upon after the corresponding stone name.

1. אַאִימַנְט—*'a'iYMaNṬ*

'a'iYMaNṬ is O. Fr. *aimant / aymant* or Angl.-Nor. *a(i)mand* meaning both 'diamond' and 'magnetite' (TL 1:240; FEW 24:132a; AND 1:9b). These two meanings are also present in our text as it mentions two variants of this stone:

דִיַאמַנְט (*DiYa'MaNṬ*) is O. Fr. / Angl.-Nor. *diamant*, 'diamond' (TL 2: 1909; FEW 24:132b; AND 2:188a); also cf. entry no. 38;

מַגְנֵיטְיש (*MaGNeYṬəYŠ*) is Lat. *magnetes* 'magnetite' (ThLL 8:104).

2. אקטץ—*'QṬṢ*

'QṬṢ is O. Fr. / Angl.-Nor. *acates*, 'agate' (TL 1:207; AND 1:16b), variant of *agate* (TL 1:206; FEW 24:103a). The Hebrew spelling corresponds to the one given in the First French Version of Marbode's Lapidary (*acates*, see FF 89); also cf. the corresponding spelling of שְׁזִילְא (*ŠəZYiLə'*), 'Sicily', and *Sezíle* in FF (92).

קַרֵיטְא (*QaReYṬə'*) should be read as O. Fr./Angl.-Nor. *Crete* (FF 100), 'Crete', with an erroneous punctuation of the first syllable.

קורָל (*QWRaL*) is O. Fr. / Angl.-Nor. *coral*, 'coral' (TL 2:843; FEW 2-2:1178a; AND 1:115a). The term also features in DB (252).

3. אַלֵיקְטוּיְינְא—*'aLeYQṬWuYəYNə'*

'aLeYQṬWuYəYNə' must be identified with O. Fr. *alectoire*, 'alectorius' (TL 1:277; FEW 24:321b). The Hebrew spelling in our text suggests a reading **alectuine* or the like. This form, however, could not be retrieved in our sources and might be corrupt (šuruq instead of ḥolem and nun instead of resh) for *alectoire*.

פיבא (*PYB'*) is O. Fr. / Angl.-Nor. *feve*, 'bean' (TL 3:1798; FEW 3:339a; AND 3:303b).

4. אֵשמַרַלְדְא—*'eŠMRaLDə'*

'eŠMRaLDə' is O. Fr. / Angl.-Nor. *esmeralde*, 'emerald' (TL 3:1117; FEW 12:9b; AND 2:263a); also cf. entry no. 39.

פורלש (*PWRLŠ*) must be the rectus singular[57] or rather the plural form of O. Fr. / Angl.-Nor. *por(r)el*, 'leek', which was normally spelled *poriaus* / *porreus* (TL 7:1502; FEW 9:194b; AND 5:541b).

שאיאה (*Š'Y'H*) must be read as Lat. *Scythia*, 'land of the Scythes' (GH 2:2554) or rather Angl.-Nor. *Cithie* with the same meaning in the CL (193); the term seems to be corrupt without a ṭet (read: *Š'ṬY'H*).

5. אוניקלא—*'WNYQL'*

'WNYQL' is O. Fr. / Angl.-Nor. *onicle*, 'onyx' (TL 6:1126; FEW 7:356b; AND 4:465b). The spelling *onicle* (variant of *oniche, onyx*, see TL loc. cit.; FEW loc. cit.) can be found especially in Angl.-Nor. lapidaries (see, e.g., VA 455; FP XLVI; SP VII).

שַׁרְדִינְא (*ŠaRDiYNə'*) is O. Fr. / Angl.-Nor. *sardine*, another name for 'sard' (TL 9:182; FEW 11:226b; AND 6:677b).

6. אִיטִיטְא—*'iYṬiṬə'*

'iYṬiṬə' is O. Fr. / Angl.-Nor. *et(h)ite*, 'aetites, eagle-stone' (TL 3:1519; FEW 24:240a; AND 2:285a). The Ms. shows a vocalization of the first syllable with [i] instead of [e]; for the oscillation between these two sounds, cf. the introduction.

אוקְצִיַאן (*'WoQṢiYa'N*) is, because of the vowelization, rather Angl.-Nor. *occian*, 'ocean, sea' (AND 4:461b) than O. Fr. *oc(c)ean*, id. (TL 6:961; FEW 7:302b).

7. אאליוטרופא—*''LYWṬRWP'*

''LYWṬRWP' is O. Fr. / Angl.-Nor. *(h)eliotrope / elyotrope*, 'heliotrope' (TL 3:32; FEW 4:398b: AND 2:206a). In O. Fr. this term designated a precious stone as well as the sunflower (cf. TL loc. cit.).

---

[57] The two-case system, however, became moribund from the middle of the 12th c. on (cf. Pope 1934:462–463).

8. אַבִּישְׁטא—*'aBiYŠṬ'*

'aBiYŠṬ' must be read as O. Fr. / Angl.-Nor. *abeste*, 'asbestos' (TL 1:559; FEW 25–1:407a; AND 1:2b). For *-i-* instead of *-e-*, cf. the introduction; also cf. entry no. 10.

9. אֵימַטִּיש—*'eYMaṬiYŠ*

'eYMaṬiYŠ must be identified with O. Fr. / Angl.-Nor. *ematite(s)*, 'hematite' (TL 3:33; FEW 4:376a; AND 2:206b). A variant with final [-s] could not be retrieved in our sources and the šin seems to be erroneous for ṭet. The Hebrew transcription suggests—because of a lacking 'alef or yod—that final [ə] was not any longer pronounced; the same suggestion is also made by other entries in the *Ko'aḥ ha-Avanim* (cf. the introduction).

קוליריו (*QWLYRYW*) belongs to Lat. *collyrium*, 'eye-salve' (MLWB 2:875; ThLL 3:1668; GH 1:1278). The lacking representation of the final nasal *-m* is a common phenomenon, which can also be found in other Latin texts in Hebrew transcription, e.g. in the *Sefer ha-Shimmush*, entry Dalet 1: *SNMWMW* for Lat. 'cinnamumum' (cf. Bos/ Mensching et al., forthcoming). This transcription reflects the actual effaced pronounciation of final *-m* in the epoch of Late Latin (cf. Pope 1934:97).

10. אַבֵּישְׁט—*'aBeYŠṬ*

'aBeYŠṬ is O. Fr. / Angl.-Nor. *abeste*, 'asbestos' (for references, cf. entry no. 8). For the pronunciation of final [ə], cf. the introduction.

11. אֵיקְשַׁקְרַטְלִיטו—*'eYQŠaQRaṬLiYṬW*

'eYQŠaQRaṬLiYṬW must be corrupt for M. Lat. *exacontalithos*, 'exacontalitus' (MLWB 3:1462 with reference to *hexacontali-*), literally 'having the colours of 60 stones'. *Hexecontalithos* (transcription of Gr. ἑξηκοντάλιθος) features, e.g., already in Pliny (nat. XXX, 167), but the identity of the stone is unknown to us (cf. ThLL 6–3:2681; GH 1:3044).

12. אוֹרֵיטא—*'WoReṬ'*

'WoReYṬ' is O. Fr. / Angl.-Nor. *orit(h)e*, 'a precious stone, oritis' (TL 6:1285; FEW 7:417a; AND 4:469b). For the oscillation between *-e-* and *-i-* in the second syllable, see the introduction.

13. אַנִידְרְא—*'aNiYDRə'*

'aNiYDRə' must be O. Fr. / Angl.-Nor. *enidre*, 'enhygros, a marvellous, water exuding stone' (TL 3:427; AND 2:229b) with initial nasal [ã] instead of [ẽ]; a confusion between these two nasal sounds can be observed often in medieval Jud.-Fr. texts, e.g., the alternation between אֵן (*en*, fol. 157a–8) and אַן (*an*, fol. 162b–16) in the anonymous medical compilation *Fevres* (ed. Zwink, unedited). However, if we presume that nasal vowels have already disappeared in this epoch of Angl.-Nor. (cf. the introduction), we deal here with a phenomenon that will often occur in this Ms, i.e., the confusion or oscillation between [a] and [e]. Vowelizations with patah instead of tsere (or the inverse case) seem to be a typical peculiarity of Lat. / Romance lexemes the *Ko'aḥ ha-Avanim* (cf. the introduction).

14. אֵימַטִישְא—*'eYMaṬiYŠə'*

'eYMaṬiYŠə', **ematice*, corresponds to O. Fr. / Angl.-Nor. *ametiste*, 'amethyst' (TL 1:349; FEW 24:436a; AND 1:25b). Initial tsere stands here instead of patah (for details, cf. the introduction). The lack of [-t-] in the last syllable can also be found in the variants *matice* and *aumatiz*, id., given in TL and FEW (loc. cit.).

פֵּישְקְש (*PeYŠQŠ*) is the plural of O. Fr. *p(i)esque*, 'peach' (TL 7:820; FEW 8:265a); the Angl.-Nor. has *pe(s)che / peiche*—variants that would match less well with our term.

אֵמַה (*'eMaH*) is Gr. ἅιμα, 'blood' (LS 38a).

צונצא גרנט (*ṢWNṢ' GRNṬ*) may correspond, with respect to a corrupt spelling of the first element, to O. Fr. *jagonce grenat*, 'garnet red jacinth' (TL 4:1537), which is, according to Marbode, the reddish variety of the hyacinthus (cf. Marb. Red. lap. XIV). Also cf. entry no. 62.

שֵׂרְדָא (*ŠeRDǝ'*) is O. Fr. / Angl.-Nor. *sarde*, 'sard, a variety of reddish chalcedony' (TL 9:181; FEW 11:226b; AND 6:677b). For the oscillation between [a] and [e] in the first syllable, cf. the introduction.

15. אַלְמְדִינְא—*'aLMDiYNǝ'*

'aLMDiYNǝ' must be read as O. Fr. / Angl.-Nor. *alemandine* (variants: *alamandine, alemandina, alabandine*) 'alabandica, a precious stone' (TL 1:282; FEW 24:287a; AND 1:20a). The lack of *-n-* (*'aLMDiYNǝ'* instead of *'aLMNDiYNǝ'*) indicates probably the disappearance of nasalization (cf. the introduction).

16. אֵינִיאַה—*'eYNiY'aH*

'eYNiY'aH is Lat. *(h)yenia*, variant of *hyaenia*, 'hyaena-stone, chelidonia' (ThLL 6–3:3130) and appears also in Angl.-Nor. texts, e.g., as *hyenia* (AL 1171) or *hienia* (FP XXXIII).

איניאה (*'YNY'H*) represents Lat. *(h)yaena* 'hyaena' (ThLL 6–3:3129; GH 1:3096).

17. אִירוֹנְא—*'iYRWoNǝ'*

The form *'iYRWoNǝ'* is difficult to analyse. The informations Berakhyah gives for this stone indicate that *iris*, O. Fr. / Angl.-Nor. for 'iris (a variety of quartz)' (TL 4:1458: FEW 4:813a; AND 3:364b) must be meant (cf. section 3). We might either suppose a corrupt spelling for, e.g., something like *'iYRYŠ*, but the fact that the term אירונא (*'YRWN'*, without punctuation) features a second time in this entry must give us cause for further research.

The form may suggest a relation to O. Fr. *aurone*, 'southernwood (Artemisia abrotanum)' (TL 1:681; FEW 24:48a) or to O. Fr. / Angl.-Nor. *irai(g)ne*, 'spider' (TL 4:1433; FEW 25–1:77b–78a; AND 3:364b), but the context requires definitively the name of stone. Actually, we find in the FEW (25–1:80b) the Mod. Fr. (18th c.) *aran(n)ea*, stemming from the same etymon as *iraine* (i.e., Lat. ARANEA), as a scientific neologism for 'minerai d'argent composé de fils d'argent' (i.e., silver mineral, composed of silver threads). We might perhaps assume that a related variant of the mentioned Mod. Fr. term, i.e., something like *iraine/ *irone*, was already used in former epochs to designate a stone, although the Mod. Fr. *aranea* seems to refer to another kind.

18. אַנְדְּרוֹ דְּרַגַּצַא—*'aNdRWo DRaGaṢa'*

'aNdRWo DRaGaṢa', **andro dragaza* or the like, seems to be corrupt and has to be identified—because of its ending with *-a-* with Lat. *androdragma*, variant of *androdamas*, 'androdamas (a sulphurous ore)' (ThLL 2:37; MLWB 1:630). In O. Fr. / Angl.-Nor., we have *androd(r)agme* (TL 1:384; FEW 24:522a; AND 1:28a).[58]

19. אופטליאש—*'WPṬLY'Š*

'WPṬLY'Š has to be identified with O. Fr. / Angl.-Nor. *optallie* 'opal' (TL 6:1159; FEW 7:358b; AND 4:466a). Our term seems either to be the plural of this word or it got blended with variants of this word conserving the final *-s* of their etymon, OPALUS, e.g. *optals* (AND loc. cit.; FF 843) or *optalius* (AL 1523).[59] A corresponding graphical variant can be found in CL (1171, *optallies*). The Hebrew letter lamed represents here probably the sound [ʎ]; cf. the introduction.

20. אַבְשִׁיטְא—*'aBŠiYṬə'*

'aBŠiYṬə' corresponds to Angl.-Nor. *absite*, variant of O. Fr. *absicte*, 'apsyctos, a stone' (TL 1:67) without *-c-*, which is also found in the Cambridge Version of Marbode (CL 1245). For the Gr.-Lat. term of this stone, *apsyctos*, cf. entry no. 24.

21. אֱלִיקְטְרוּם—*'eLiYQṬRWM*

'eLiYQṬRWM is Lat. *electrum*, 'sucinum, genus resinae praetiosae in lapidem duratae (amber)' (ThLL 5-2:331; MLWB 3:1166). For the confusion between *-e-* and *-i-*, cf. the introduction.

22. אֻופטלוּש—*'uWPṬLWuŠ*

'uWPṬLWuŠ must be related to Late Lat. *optallius* (variant of *opalus* or *opallius*, documented, e.g., in Damigeron XXIV, ed. Abel), 'opal'

[58] The vocalization of the final syllable with patah does not necessarily admit the conclusion of a Lat. word (cf. entries nos. 20, 55, 56, and 65, where patah represents probably final sheva), but Lat. should be the first language to be taken into consideration.

[59] The *-t-* in the derivations is due to the influence of the Gr. ὀφθαλμός, 'eye' (cf. FEW loc. cit.).

(ThLL 9–2:659). The initial vocalisation with *u-* suggested by the Ms. (**uptalus* or the like) seems to be erroneous. For further discussion cf. entry no. 19.

23. אֲנְקוֹטְרא—*'aNQWṬR'*

The term *'aNQWṬR'* could not be definitely identified. Perhaps the *acintota* is meant, which features in Meyer's edition of the Lat. abridgement of the AL (cf. Meyer 1909:549; also cf. section 3, no. 23) and features in the AL as *jacinctizonta* (AL 1293). It is taken from Isidore (Isid. nat. orig. XVI, 9, 3: *iacinthizonta*), where it is identified with the *iacinthum*, 'hyacinthe'.

24. אֲסִצְטוּש—*'aSiṢṬWoŠ*

'aSiṢṬWoŠ could not be identified with absolute certainty, but reminds us of Lat. *apsyctus* (M. Lat. *absictus*) 'gemma quaedam nigra' (ThLL 2:323; MLWB 1:48). For the O. Fr. term cf. entry no. 20.

25. אֲנְסְרַא—*'aNSRa'*

The term *'aNSRa'* must refer to what is called in M. Lat. texts *ambra* 'excrementa piscis, ambergis' (MLWB 1:549). It designates the waxy grey substance secreted by the intestinal lining of the sperm whale and features, e.g., in the *Sefer ha-Shimmush* as **אנברא**.[60] Our term seems to be corrupt with samech instead of bet.

בַלֵינְא (*BaLeYNə'*) is O. Fr. / Angl.-Nor *baleine/ balaine/ balenie*, 'whale' (TL 1:815; FEW 1:222b; AND 1:60b).

26. אֵישְׁטְרִיטַש—*'eYŠiṬRiYṬaŠ*

'eYŠiṬRiYṬaŠ must be identified with Lat. *ast(e)rites*, 'gemma', probably 'chatoyant' (ThLL 2:949; GH 1:656). The first syllable is vocalized with [e] instead of [a]; the last one presents the inverse case. The confusion between these two vowels can also be found in other terms of this Ms.; for this phenomenon, cf. the introduction.

60 Cf. Bos & Mensching (2001:26–27); Bos/ Mensching et al. (forthcoming, Alef no. 1).

27. אַמַאְונְטְש—*'aMa'uWNṬŠ*

aMa'uWNṬŠ might either correspond to Lat. *amiantus*, 'lapis, kind of asbestos' (ThLL 1:1889; GH 1:377) or to Fr. *amiantes* (plural of *amiante*) in the same meaning, but note that this term is only documented for M. Fr. (cf. FEW 24:437a) and that a plural form would be unusual in our context. However, the Hebrew vocalisation of the second syllable must be erroneous.

28. בֵּיֵרֵיל—*BeYReYL*

BeYReYL is O. Fr. / Angl.-Nor. *beril*, 'beryl' (TL 1:928; FEW 1:339b; AND 1:67a). For the oscillation between *-e-* and *-i-*, cf. the introduction.

29. גְּרִיזוּלֵיט—*GRiYZWLeYṬ*

GRiYZWLeYṬ is O. Fr. / Angl.-Nor. *grisolite* (variant of *crisolite*), 'chrysolite' (TL 2:1063; FEW 2–1:659a; AND 1:123b). For the oscillation between *-e-* and *-i-*, cf. the introduction; for the pronunciation of final [ə], which is not transcribed in the Hebrew term, cf. the introduction.

30. גְּרִיזוֹפְּרְש—*GRiYZoWPRŠ*

GRiYZoWPRŠ is O. Fr. / Angl.-Nor. *grisop(r)ase* (variant of *crisopace*), 'chrysoprase, a yellow-viridescent topaz' (TL 2:1064; FEW 2–1:659a; AND 3:343a). The vocalisation of the final syllable seems to be erroneous for *-PRaŠ*. For the pronunciation of final [ə], cf. the introduction. Also cf. the following entry no. 31.

The form אוירטץ (*'WYRṬṢ*) corresponds, at first sight, to the plural of O. Fr. / Angl.-Nor. *orte(i)l*, 'toe' (TL 6:1314; FEW 25–1:376b; AND 4:470a), i.e. *ortiz* (AND loc. cit.). The context of the *Ko'aḥ ha-Avanim*, indeed, suggests a kind of disease. We might possibly think of Angl.-Nor. *(gute) artetice*, 'gout' (AND 1:40a; FEW 25–1:370a), admitting that the spelling does not match perfectly: initial *'WY-* does usually not represent [a-],[61] and, moreover, a second *-Ṭ-* would be lacking.

[61] The representation of [-o], as assumed in the hypothesis of *ortiz*, is also somewhat problematic, since *-'W-* alone would be sufficient, and *-Y-* remains unexplained.

31. גרישופציאון—*GRYŠWPṢY'WN*

GRYŠWPṢY'WN corresponds to M. Lat. *crisopacion* (variant of Lat. *chrysoprasus*),[62] 'species gemmae' (MLWB 2:561). This term designates the same stone as the one discussed in entry no. 30. The name results, according to MLWB (loc. cit.), from a blend between χρυσόπρασος and τοπάζιον and features, e.g., in Marbode (Marb. Red. Lap. LX). The initial gimmel in our text seems to be an analogy to the initial Gimmel in *grisopras* (see entry no. 30).

32. גַגַטרֹום—*GaGaṬRoWM*

GaGaṬRoWM corresponds somehow to O. Fr. / Angl.-Nor. *gagatromé/ gagatromee* (var.: *-tromeo, -tromen, -tromeu, -troenes*) (TL 4:27; FEW 4:21b; AND 3:325b), which are loanwords of Lat. *gagatromeus*. A form without final [-e], as suggested in our Ms., could not be found. The stone is mentioned in Damigeron (Damig. lap. XLI: *gagatromanes*) and also appears in Marbode (Marb. Red. lap. XXVII: *gagatromeum*) and Albertus Magnus (*gagatronica*, Albert. M. miner. II, 2, 7). Its identity is unclear ("nomen lapidis orig. inc.", ThLL 6–2:1669; also cf. Riddle 65); perhaps it is entirely fabulous (cf. Wyckoff 94).

33. גַלַקְטִיטַש—*GaLaQṬiYṬaŠ*

GaLaQṬiYṬaŠ is Lat. *galactites*, 'galactite, a stone' (ThLL 6–2:1669). The punctuation with patah instead of sheva in the last syllable seems to be, at first sight, erroneous. But the same phenomenon can also be found in other Lat. and Romance lexemes of the *Ko'aḥ ha-Avanim*, so that a simple qualification of corruption would not be satisfactory. This uncommon representation of *-e-* might rather indicate a quite open and frontal pronunciation of the schwa sound (cf. the introduction).

34. גַלִיקְטוֹטְיַא—*GaLiQṬWoṬYa'*

The term *GaLiQṬWoṬYa'* could not be identified. Perhaps we have to think of a Romance derivation from Lat. *chalcitis*, 'ore; green vitriol; melanterit' (ThLL 3:984; MLWB 2:511), whose colour is green as

[62] Featuring, e.g., in Plin. nat. XXXVII, 77.

described in the text. Or is it a (corrupt) variant of the previous stone, the green *galactites*?

35. גְלַקְצִיאַשׁ—*GLaQṢiY'aŠ*

GLaQṢiY'aŠ corresponds to M. Lat. *gelazias*, 'chalazia, hailstone' (MLWB 2:510), variant of (M.) Lat. *chalazias* (ThLL 3:983; MLWB, loc. cit.). Marbode has *galatia* (Marb. Red. lap. XXXVII). The term entered O. Fr. as *gelace, galacias, galatias* and *gelange* (Studer & Evans 399). The presence of -*Q*- is erroneous. Also cf. entry no. 44.

36. דיאַדְקוּדְא—*DY'aDQWDə'*

DY'aDQWDə' is O. Fr. / Angl.-Nor. *diadocode* (var.: *diadocos, diacodus*) 'diadocos, a stone' (TL 2:1907; AND 2:188a).

37. דְאוֹנִישׁ—*Də'oWNiYŠ*

Də'oWNiYŠ is O. Fr. / Angl.-Nor. *dionise*, 'dionysia, a stone' (TL 2:1932; AND 2:189b). For the oscillation between -*e*- and -*i*- in the Hebrew graphical representation, cf. the introduction. For the pronunciation of final [ə], cf. the introduction.

38. דִיאַמַנְט—*DiY'aMaNṬ*

DiY'aMaNṬ is O. Fr. / Angl.-Nor. *diamant*, 'diamond' (TL 2:1909; FEW 24:133a; AND 2:188a). This term was often used for 'magnet, load-stone' (cf. Studer & Evans 393). Also cf. entry no. 1, where Berakhyah mentions the *diamant* as a variety of the *aimant*. This entry treats the *diamant* in its property of attracting iron separately.

אַצִיר (*'aṢiYR*) is Angl.-Nor. *ascir*, 'steel' (documented only in the online version of the AND).[63] We might exclude an O. Fr. word here, since for O. Fr., we could only find diphthongized forms like *acier* (TL 1:86b; FEW 24:104b).

[63] See URL: http://www.anglo-norman.net/gate/ s.v. *acer* (31/10/2007).

39. טֹורְקְוִיש—*ṬoWRQWiYŠ*

ṬoWRQWiYŠ must be read as O. Fr. *turquois* or Angl.-Nor. *turkoise* 'turquoise' (TL 10:727; FEW 19:190b; AND 7:843a). The vocalisation of the first syllable seems to result from an uncertainty to represent the phone [y] with Hebrew characters.

אשמרלדא (*'ŠMRLD'*) is O. Fr. *esmeralde*, 'emerald'; cf. entry no. 4.

וינש (*WYNŠ*) is the plural of Angl.-Nor. *vene*, 'vein' (AND 7:849b). This term rather suggests to be, due to the simple *-Y-*, the explicite Angl.-Nor. *vene* and less the diphthongized form *veine*, which was the common variant in O. Fr. (cf. TL 11:139; FEW 14:226a).

גֵייטְא (*GeYYṬ'ə*) is O. Fr. *jaiet* / Angl.-Nor. *gaiet* / *gagate*, 'jet' (TL 4:1544; FEW 4:21a; AND 3:325b). For the vocalization of the first syllable with [e] instead of [a] and further discussion, cf. the introduction and the main entry no. 42.

40. טֹופַסְא—*ṬoWPaSə'*

ṬoWPaSə' is O. Fr. / Angl.-Nor. *t(h)opace* / *topasse* / *topaze*, 'topaz' (TL 10:385; FEW 13-2:35b; AND 7:799b).

41. יַשְׁפְא—*YaŠPə'*

YaŠPə' is O. Fr. / Angl.-Nor. *jaspe*, 'jasper' (TL 4:1594; FEW 5:32a; AND 3:368a).

42. יאייט—*Y'YYṬ*

Y'YYṬ is O. Fr. *jaiet* / *gaiet* or Angl.-Nor. *gaiet*, 'jet' (TL 4:1544; FEW 4:21a; AND 3:325b), hailing from Lat. GAGATES (FEW loc. cit.). Lat. GA- became [ʒɑ]—via [ʤɑ]—in O. Fr. and was represented in the Lat. alphabet by the letters <ja>.[64] The initial Yod probably represents here the O. Fr. phone [ʒ] (rather than [ʤ], cf. the introduction); also cf. entry no. 39.

[64] Cf. Rheinfelder 1963:164; 167.

43. יַרַייִטא—*YaRaYiYṬ'*

YaRaYiYṬ' has to be identified with O. Fr. / Angl.-Nor. *gerachite*, 'hieracitis'[65] (TL 4:282; FEW 4:426a; AND 3:334a). For the Yod representing the sound [ʒ] and the oscillation between [a] and [e], cf. the introduction.

44. יִילַצַא—*YiYLaṢa'*

YiYLaṢa' corresponds to M. Lat. *gelazia*, 'chalazia, hailstone'; for references and further discussion, see entry no. 35. For Yod representing the sound [ʒ] at the beginning of a syllable and the oscillation between [e] and [i] in the initial syllable, cf. the introduction. A variant without an *-i-* in the final syllable, suggested by the Ms. (**gelaza* or the like), is not attested.

גרזייל (*GRZYL*) is O. Fr. / Angl.-Nor. *gresil(le)*, 'hail' (TL 4:626; FEW 16:85b; AND 3:342a).

45. לְיְנֵיטְא—*LəYNeYṬə'*

LəYNeYṬə' represents possibly a non-documented O. Fr. loan word **legnete* or the like, modelled upon the Lat. basis *lignita* (variant of the more common *lychnites*, see ThLL 7:1939; also cf. Damigeron lap. XXVIII),[66] and refers to a stone called otherwise *lychnis* in Lat. texts (Plin. nat. XXXVII, 103; Isid. ety. XVI,14,4). Alternatively, but less probably in our opinion, Lat. *lignita* itself could be represented, if we consider the particular transcribing conventions of this Ms., especially the oscillations between *-a-* and *-e-* and between *-e-* and *-i-* (cf. the introduction). Possibly, the violet-red and rose-red tourmaline is meant (cf. the edition). The term does not feature in Marbode and the Angl.-Nor. Marbode tradition.

46. לִיגוֹרֵיאַה—*LiYGoWReY'aH*

LiYGoWReY'aH corresponds—considering the already known particularities of vowelization of our Ms., i.e. the oscillation between *-e-* and *-i-* as well as between *-a-* and *-e-*, to O. Fr. / Angl.-Nor. *ligur(i)e* (var.:

[65] Possibly arsenic ore (cf. Wyckoff 1976:95).

[66] Albert. M. min., II,2,20, has *zigrites*.

liguire). The dictionaries do not give a special meaning of this stone (cf. TL 5:455; FEW 5:482b; AND 3:388a), but in M. Lat., *ligurius* is amber (cf. Riddle 62; also cf. entry no. 21). In Latin, the amber was originally called *lyncurium* (related to *lynx*), but this term was transformed into *ligurius* in the 4th c. (cf. FEW loc. cit.), which is the etymological basis of the Romance derivations.

דֵּיטְא (*DeYṬə'*) is *date*, 'urine' (AND 2:140b; FEW 21:318b; TL 2:1198). The word features only in Angl.-Nor. texts and goes back to an uncertain origin (cf. FEW loc. cit.). For the confusion between *-a-* and *-e-*, cf. the introduction.

47. מֵידו—*MeYDW*

MeYDW must be related to M. Lat. *medus*, a term designating a stone "from Media", which was probably a mixture of impure metallic sulphates (cf. Riddle 1977:73). It features in Marbode (Marb. Red. lap. XXXVI) and entered also in Angl.-Nor. texts (cf. Studer & Evans 1924:400, beneath *mede*); Damigeron (Damig. lap. XXI) and Albertus Magnus (Albert. M. miner. II, 2, 11) have *medius*. The term is missing in the dictionaries.

48. פֵּירְלְא—*PeYRLə'*

PeYRLə' is O. Fr. / Angl.-Nor. *perle*, 'pearl' (TL 7:762; FEW 8:253b; AND 5:518b).

מרגריטא (*MRGRYṬ'*) is O. Fr. / Angl.-Nor. *margarite*, 'pearl' (TL 5:1163; FEW 6:323a; AND 4:407b).

49. פַּנְטֵירַא—*PaNṬeYRa'*

PaNṬeYRa' corresponds to M. Lat. *pantera*, 'panther stone', featuring, e.g., in Thomas Cantimpratensis (see MJE 233), a variety of the more common *pantheros* (cf. Marbode LI; Bartholomaeus Anglicus XVI, quoted from Wyckoff 1976:111) or *pantherus* (Albert. M. miner. II, 2, 14; Arnoldus Saxo, quoted from Wyckoff loc. cit.). The correct Gr.-Lat. name was *panchrus* (<Gr. πάγχρους for 'all colours'; cf. Plin. nat. XXXVII, 66, 178; Isid. nat. orig. XVI, 12, 1); the connection with the panther, a coloured animal, goes back to Damigeron and Marbode (cf. Wyckoff loc. cit.). Alternatively, we might think of the O. Fr. / Angl.-Nor. *pant(h)ere* (TL 7:135; FEW 7:569b; AND 5:488b) with final vocalisation with patah

instead of sheva, as already often occurred in the *Ko'aḥ ha-Avanim* (cf. the introduction).

Berakhyah relates the stone to a kind of jasper, as does the Second Prose Lapidary (SP 33), an early Angl.-Nor. version of Marbode, as well; the description of its supposed virtues, indeed, reminds rather of the opal (cf. Wyckoff loc. cit.; Riddle 1977:85).

50. פִּידוֹרַטַשׁ—*PiYDWoRaṬaŠ*

PiYDWoRaṬaŠ is Angl.-Nor. *pedoretes* (< Gr.-Lat. παιδέρως / PAEDEROS, cf. entry no. 51), 'paederos, a stone' (AND 5:509b). It features in the Cambridge Version of Marbode (CL 1367) and is an addition to Marbode's Lapidary. The source of the CL is unclear (not Pliny / Isidore, cf. entry no. 51). Concerning the Hebrew transcription, we observe the frequent peculiarity of punctuation in this Ms., i.e., [i] instead of [e] in the first and [a] instead of [e], in last two syllables (cf. the introduction).

51. פַּיְיטוֹרוֹשׁ—*PaYəYṬoWRoWŠ*

This stone could not be identified. The term reminds us of Lat. *paederos*, featuring in Pliny as a kind of opal (Plin. nat. XXXVII, 84) or of amethyst (Plin. nat. XXXVII, 123; cf. GH 2:1433), but the ascribed aspect and virtues in Berakhyah and in Pliny do not correspond. Isidore (nat. orig. XIV, 10) has a white *paedroros*, but mentions other virtues. For the Angl.-Nor. derivation, cf. no. 50.

52. פְּרִיטוֹרַא—*PRiYṬoWRa'*

The term *PRiYṬoWRa'* could not be identified. We might suppose a relation to the green peridot, also referred to as *olivine*, a magnesium iron silicate, which is also documented in O. Fr. as *peridot / peritot* (TL 7:749). Or do we have to suppose a relation with O. Fr. / Angl.-Nor. *pyrite / perite*, 'pyrite' (FEW 9:647b; AND 5:518b)?

גוטא קרנפא (*GWṬ' QRNP'*) is O. Fr. *gote crampe* 'gout that contracts the extremities' (TL 2:1010; FEW 16:353b, here attested only for M. Fr.). The nasalization of the [ã] in *crampe* is here indicated by a following *-n-*, and not by *-m-*, as usual in Lat. alphabet based othography. This compound term is not attested in Angl.-Nor. For *crampe*, also cf. entry no. 64.

53. קַרְבּוֹקְלא—*QaRBoWQL'*

QaRBoWQL' is O. Fr. / Angl.-Nor. *c(h)arboncle / c(h)arbuncle / charbo(u)cle*, 'carbuncle, ruby' (TL 2:256; FEW 2–1:360a; AND 1:91a), here again with lacking nasalization of the internal [-o-] (cf. the introduction). The Lat. CARBUNCULUS, etymon of the Romance forms, designates since Pliny the ruby; it is a translation of the Gr. ἄνθραξ. In the Middle Ages, the term was used to denote brilliant red stones, particularly the ruby and the garnet (cf. FEW 2–1:361a; Riddle 1977:61; Wyckoff 1976:77).

רובין (*RWBYN*) is O. Fr. *robin* / Angl.-Nor. *rubin* 'ruby, carbunculus' (TL 8:1528; FEW 10:535b; AND 6:664a). Also cf. entry no. 61.

54. קוֹרַל—*QoWRaL*

QoWRaL is O. Fr. / Angl.-Nor. *coral(e) / cural*, 'coral' (TL 2:843, no. 1; FEW 2–2:1178a; AND 1:115a, no. 1). Also cf. entry no. 2.

55. קוֹלֵירַא—*QoWLeYRa'*

QoWLeYRa' has to be read as Angl.-Nor. *colire*, 'collyria, a miraculous stone' (TL 2:567, no. 1; AND 1:105a, no. 2). The identity of the stone is uncertain. It features in the AL (665) and in (M.) Lat. texts as *collurus* (Damig. lap. XXXVIII; MJE 198) and *collire* (MJE 222). For the oscillation between *-e-* and *-i-*, as well as for the punctuation of the final syllable with patah instead of sheva, cf. the introduction.

56. קוֹרְטוֹלִינַא—*QoWRṬoWLiYNa'*

QoWRṬoWLiYNa' has to be identified with O. Fr. / Angl.-Nor. *cornoligne / cornel(l)i(g)ne / cornaline*, 'cornelian; a kind of agate' (TL 2:874; FEW 2–2:1198b; AND 1:116a). The Hebrew spelling with ṭet instead of nun must be erroneous. Nun introducing the last syllable represents here probably the sound [ɲ] (cf. the introduction). For the vocalization of the final syllable with [a] instead of [ə], cf. the introduction.

57. קְרִישְׁטַל—*QRiYŠṬaL*

QRiYŠṬaL is O. Fr. / Angl.-Nor. *cristal*, 'crystal' (TL 2:1064; FEW 2–2:13485b; AND 1:123b).

58. קַלְצִידוֹנְיַא—*QaLṢiYDoWNYa'*

QaLṢiYDoWNYa' is Lat. *calcidonia* (sc. *gemma*), 'chalcedony', a variant of *c(h)alcedonius* (MLWB 2:511). The feminine noun was the basis for the Romance derivations like O. Fr. / Angl.-Nor. *c(h)alcedoine / calcidoine* (TL 2:14; FEW 2-1:619a; AND 1:80b).

59. קַמַהוּ—*QaMaHWu*

QaMaHWu must be identified with O. Fr. / Angl.-Nor. *cama(h)ieu*, 'cameo' (TL 2:17; FEW 2-1:110b). The stone is not mentioned in Marbode, but features in the Angl.-Nor. Alphabetical Lapidary as *cachmahief* (AL 649). In Lat. texts, we find *kacamon* (Albert. M. min. II, 2, 9), *kauman* (Arnoldus Saxo, quoted from Wyckoff 1976:101) and *kamen* (Bartholomaeus Anglicus, quoted from Wyckoff loc. cit.).

60. קַלקוּפִינְא—*QaLQWPiNə'*

QaLQWPiNə' corresponds to O. Fr. *calcofone* (TL 2:15) or Angl.-Nor. *calcofonie* (FEW 2-1:619b; CL 1253) in the meaning 'chalcophonos'. Variants with internal [-fi-] could not be found; the vocalization of this syllable might thus be erroneous.

61. רוֹבִין—*RoWbiYN*

RoWbiYN corresponds to O. Fr. *robin*, 'ruby, carbunculus' (TL 8:1528; FEW 10:535b). In other Angl.-Nor. texts, we have only *rubin* (AND 6:664a) with *-u-*. Also cf. entry no. 53.

62. שפיר—*ŠPYR*

ŠPYR is O. Fr. / Angl.-Nor. *saphir(e) / safir(e)*, 'sapphire' (TL 9:39; 9:41; FEW 12:213a; AND 6:677a).

שפיר יַכַנְט (*ŠPYR YaKaNṬ*), שפיר יכַנְט (*ŠPYR YKaNṬ*), and שפיר יַכְנט (*ŠPYR YaKNṬ*) represent a non-documented compound O. Fr. / Angl.-Nor. term **saphir jacint* (with an erroneous punctuation of the last syllable in the first two variants; a variant with *-ca-*, as suggested by the Ms., is not documented in our sources), which probably refers to the same stone as O. Fr. *jargunce saphire*, "saphir qui ressemble à l'hyacinthe" (i.e., sapphire that resembles the jacinth) (FEW 4:520b). *Jargunce / jagonce* is another word for the jacinth in O. Fr. and Angl.-Nor. (cf. TL 4:1537; FEW loc. cit.; AND 3:367b). For *saphir*, cf. above. For *jacint* cf. TL (4:1528); FEW (loc. cit.); AND (3:367a);

Berakhyah mentions the jacinth as a variety of the sapphire. Confusions between these two stones can often be found in medieval lapidaries: Solinus (coll. XXX, 32, quoted from Wyckoff 1976:97), e.g., meant by his description of the *hyacinthus* probably the transparent sapphire (cf. Wyckoff loc. cit.); Albertus Magnus has two kinds of *hyacinthus*: the *aquaticus* and the *saphirinus* (Albert. M. miner. II, 2, 8), but notes in the same passage that "the jacinth is sometimes called sapphire" (Albert. M. loc. cit.).

וַוְשֶׁר שפיר (*WaWŠR ŠPYR*) is, according to our author, another variety of the sapphire. A corresponding term—something like **wazzer saphir*—could not be found in our sources. Probably, the same stone as *jagunce evage* (TL 9:41), literally 'watery jacinth', is meant, which Berakhyah treats below. The *hyacinthus aquaticus* is also discussed by Albertus Magnus (miner. II, 2, 8) and is identified by the editor as "iolite, a pale blue or violet variety of cordierite" (Wyckoff 98).

The identification of the first element of our term remains unclear—should we really suppose a Western Germanic, e.g. Old/ Middle High German, *wazzer*, 'water' (Lexer 489c; ODEE 944a)?[67] This would be the only case (beneath the variant below in this entry) in which we find a Germanic word in Berakhyah's text. We might also take in condsideration that *WaWŠR* could be a corrupt spelling of an O. Fr. / Angl.-Nor. term designating 'watery', like *evage, e(a)wer*, *yauver*, among others (TL 3:1524; AND 2:286a).

שפיר אוריאנט (*ŠPYR 'WRY'NṬ*) represents a non-documented **saphir orient*, literally 'sapphire of the orient / of the east' (O. Fr. genitive construction);[68] for *saphir*, cf. above; for O. Fr. / Angl.-Nor. *orient*, cf. TL (6:1270); FEW (7:413a); AND (4:469b). This variety of sapphire features, e.g., in the Third Prose Lapidary: "Et une maniere en troeve l'oun en Turquie, et sont apelé oriental." (i.e., and another variety can be found in Turkey, and they are called *oriental*.) (TP III). Marbode (Marb. Red. lap. V) and Albertus Magnus (miner. II, 2, 17) treat a kind of sapphire that comes from the east (*Media* in Marbode and *India* in Albert. M.), but they give another name: *sirtites*.

---

[67] In O. Engl., only *wæter* with intervocalic [-t-] is attested (cf. ODEE loc. cit.).

[68] Cf. Rheinfelder 1967:42.

מילפוייל (*MYLPWYYL*) is O. Fr. / Angl.-Nor. *milfoil*, 'yarrow (Achillea millefolium)' (TL 6:47; FEW 6–2:92b; AND 4:427a).

For יָכַנְט (*YaKaNṬ*) and יכנט (*YKNṬ*), *jacint*, cf. above.

יסיטא (*YSYṬ'*) must be identified again, in our opinion, with O. Fr. / Angl.-Nor. *jacinte* (for references, cf. above). We have here a variant not representing the *-n-*, which might either indicate that [n] of the nasal [ɛ̃n] was no longer pronounced, or—more probably—that nazalisation on the whole was in course of disappearance at this epoch of Angl.-Nor. (cf. the introduction).

Berakhyah mistakenly takes it for a variety of the jacinth mentioned above, which is, for its part, divided into three kinds. In the Marbode tradition the jacinth also has three varieties, but there they are named *granati, citrini* and *veneti* (Marb. Red. lap. XIV).

For טופסא (*ṬWPS'*), *topace*, cf. entry no. 40.

ושר יכנט (*WŠR YKNṬ*) must refer to the 'water jacinth'. We have here an unidentified element *WŠR*, which is similar to *WaWŠR* in this entry above. *WŠR* again might represent a Germanic term for 'water' (for references, cf. above). For the second element *YKNṬ*, cf. above.

This second (third in Marbode) variety of the jacinth, called *venetus* in Marbode (cf. above) is designated *euage* (FF 344) / *ewage* (FP X) or *ewagine* (VA 365) in the Angl.-Nor. Marbode tradition.

For קרישטל (*QRYŠṬL*), *cristal*, cf. entry no. 57.

עלישטרא (*'LYŠṬR'*) is, according to Berakhyah, the third variant of the *jacint*. A corresponding term could not be found in our sources and must remain unexplained.

יגונצא מרינא (*YGWNṢ' MRYN'*) is O. Fr. / Angl.-Nor. **jagonce marine*, literally 'marine jacinth'. The combination of these two elements could not be found in our sources, but Berakhyah seems here again to mean the 'watery jacinth' (cf. above), i.e. the third variety of the jacinth in Marbode. For *jagonce*, see above; for *marin, -e*, cf. TL (5:1173); FEW (6–1:344b); AND (4:407b).

יכנט גרנט (*YKNṬ GRNṬ*) is O. Fr. **jacint grenat*, literally 'garnet red jacinth'. For *jacinth*, cf. above; for *grenat*, cf. TL (4:615); FEW (4:238a). Since *jacint* is another word for *jagonce* (see above), our term must refer to the same stone as *jagonce grenat* (TL 4:1537) and is thus the first variety of the *hyacinthus*, the *granatus*, mentioned in Marbode (loc. cit.). Also cf. entry no. 14.

63. שׂוּלְנִיטֵי—*ŠoWLNiYṬeY*

ŠoWLNiYṬeY is *solenite*, 'selenite, moonstone' (AND 6:711). This term (with the more common variants *silenite / selenite*, see TL 9:656; FEW 11:415b; AND loc. cit.) is only documented in Angl.-Nor. texts.

64. שַׂרְדִינְא—*ŠaRdiYNə'*

ŠaRdiYNə' is O. Fr. *sardine*—another name for *sarde*—'sard' (TL 9:182; FEW 11:226b).

קרנפא (*QRNP'*) is O. Fr. / Angl.-Nor. *crampe*, 'cramp; tetanus' (TL 2:1011; FEW 16:354a; AND 1:121a). Just like in entry no. 52 (*gote crampe*), the nasalization of the [a] in *crampe* is here indicated by nun, and not by mem.

65. שַׂרְדַא אוֹנִיקָא—*ŠaRDa' 'oWNiYQa'*

ŠaRDa' 'oWNiYQa' seems to be at first sight Lat.—due to its endings in *-a-* but a corresponding variant could not be found in our sources, where we have only *sardonyx / sardonychus/ -a* (GH 2:2493; LTL 4:225c) or the simple lexemes *sardius* (GH 2:2492; LTL 4:225b) and *onyx* (GH 2:1351; ThLL 9–2:654). We might also assume a—less verisimilar—ad hoc combination of Lat. *sarda* 'a gemstone' (the masculine kind is our sard, the feminine our cornelian, cf. GH 2:2491; LTL 4:225a) and a non attested **onyca*. It seems rather probable to us that we deal here with a (non documented) variant of O. Fr. / Angl.-Nor. *sardonixe / sardonice*, 'sardonyx, a form of onyx' (TL 9:183; FEW 11:229a; AND 6:677b). If we admit a punctuation with patah instead of sheva in the final syllables, as already often occured in this edition (cf. the introduction), we would get something like **sarde onique*, which is quite similar to the Romance forms.

66. שרפנטינא—*ŠRPNṬYN'*

ŠRPNṬYN' corresponds to O. Fr. *serpentine*, 'a gem stone; snake stone' (TL 9:543). The stone is neither described in the Marbode tradition nor in its precursors. The term *serpentine* (as a stone) features in a poem of

Rutebeuf (1235–1285, Paris)[69] and is identified with the *pantere* (panther stone, cf. entry no. 49) in the Angl.-Nor. Verse Adaption (VA 297) without being specially treated.

67. שדד—*ŠDD*

ŠDD is probably O. Fr. / Angl.-Nor. *sad(d)e*, 'sagda; barnacle shells' (TL 9:181; AND 6:669b). Although *sade* features in the FEW as a variant of O. Fr. *sarde* (FEW 11:226b), they must be distinguished according to Marbode, who treats them—as well as his Angl.-Nor. literary successors—seperately. The *sard* is, according to this, described as a (dark) red stone (cf. Marb. Red. lap. X) and is today a variety of reddish chalcedony or of carnelian (cf. Riddle 1977:48), whereas the *sadda* attaches itself to to ships (cf. Marb. Red. lap. XXXV; CL XXXIV) and is identified today with barnacle.

פרימא (*PRYM'*) is O. Fr. / Angl.-Nor. *pra(s)me*, 'prase (a green stone)' (TL 7:1694; FEW 9:329a; AND 5:545b).

68. תרשיש—*TRŠYŠ*

TRŠYŠ is a Hebrew term (possibly our aquamarine, cf. the edition of the Ms.).

צירוניא (*ṢYRWNY'*) is O. Fr. / Angl.-Nor. *ceraune / cheronne*, 'ceraunius, thunder-stone' (TL 2:119; AND 1:85a). Also cf. entry no. 72.

71. צִילִידוֹנְיָא—*ṢiYLiYDoWNYa'*

ṢiYLiYDoWNYa' is *cilidonia*, a M. Lat. variant of Lat. *chelidonia*, 'chelidony' (MLWB 2:531; ThLL 3:1004).

אֲרַדנלא (*'aRaDNL'*) must be identified with O. Fr. *arondel(l)e* / Angl.-Nor. *arundele* '(little) swallow' (TL 1:543; FEW 4:434b; FF 396, among others). The Hebrew spelling contains a metathesis (*-nd-* > *-dn-*); the second syllable is vocalized with [a]: corresponding (modern) variants like *arandela, arandale* could only be found for the Francoprovençal spoken region and for Burgundy (cf. FEW loc. cit.), so that we suppose an erroneous punctuation for our north-eastern French text.

---

69 Quoted in TL, loc. cit.

צִיפַרְשׁ (*ṢiYPRaŠ*) is O. Fr. / Angl.-Nor. *cipres*, 'cypress (Cypressus sempervirens)' (TL 2:438; FEW 2–2:1613a; AND 1:99a) with a vocalization with patah instead of tsere in the final syllable (cf. the introduction).

72. צֵירִיאוֹן—*ṢeYRiY'oWN*

ṢeYRiY'oWN must be identified with O. Fr. / Angl.-Nor. *ceraune* / *cheronne*, 'ceraunius, thunder-stone' (TL 2:119; AND 1:85a). The vocalization of the second syllable with *-i-* must be erroneous; final [-ə] is not represented by the Hebrew spelling, which indicates an inconsistent pronounciation of this sound (cf. the introduction).

3. *Berakhyah's Sources*

The following section presents a detailed source analysis for every single stone. The information about the virtue, origin and physical aspect of the stone is traced back to the source texts that Berakhyah has probably used; striking literal parallels in Latin and Anglo-Norman lapidaries are quoted and translated by the author. The abbreviations of the source texts are explained when they occur for the first time; moreover, they feature in the bibliography.

1. *aimant*

The confusion of terms for the *aimant* (*adamas* in Lat.)—the *diamant* and the *magnetes* are treated as varieties of the *aimant*—dates back at least to Pliny the Elder (Plin. nat.[70] XXXVII, 55–61); it is also present in Marbode and remains in the medieval translations. Marbode mentions four varieties of this stone (as does Berakhyah): 1. a hard variety (the diamond) hailing from India; 2. a second variant from Arabia; 3. a third variety from Cyprus; 4. the magnetite; the key to this identification is the assertion that the fourth variety of *adamas* attracts iron (cf. Marb. Red. lap.[71] I, 24–49).

The Angl.-Nor. Cambridge Version of Marbode's Lapidary[72] (CL) is Berakhyah's main source for the *aimant*, but we also find close parallels to

[70] Gaius Plinius Secundus, *Naturalis Historia*, ed. and transl. König (1979).
[71] Marbodus Redonensis, *De lapidibus*, ed. Riddle (1977).
[72] *The Cambridge Version of Marbode's Lapidary*, ed. Studer & Evans (1924).

the Angl.-Nor. First and Second Prose Versions[73] (FP and SP). From the CL he took the information about the place where the *aimant* is found: *They are found in mines of gold, silver and copper* → "Kar il les trovent enz es mines / La u l'en trove les metals, / L'or, le quivre, les cristals" (Because you find it in the mines, there, where you find the metals, gold, copper and cristal.) (CL 6–8).

The virtue of the *magnete* of attracting iron and the difference to the *diamant*, which takes the needle away goes also back to the CL: *The magnete stone, which belongs to this variety, is known to attract iron. But the diamant, because of its superior force, takes the needle away from it* → "D'aïmant quarte manire / [...] Une force ces pieres unt / De traire fer; pareilles sunt / Magnete: le fer traire solt, / Mais li daïmant li tolt" (A fourth variety of *aïmant* [...]. The stones have the power to attract iron; similar is the *magnete*: it attracts iron, but the *daïmant* neutralizes it.) (CL 37–40). The information that the stone is used by magicians, that it brings dreamless sleeps, and that it protects its owner from his enemies is also borrowed form the Cambridge Lapidary (cf. CL 41–48).

For the power of this stone to help the seamen to take the right sailing direction, the SP seems to be the source: *There is one variety of it which the seamen carry with them, because owing to it they know, when they drift on the sea, which way leads in the right direction [...]* → "E par ceste pere et par sa grant vertu cunuysent li mariners les venz" (And by this stone and by its great power, the seamen know the direction.) (SP XVIII). The FP has a closer wording concerning the place on the body where it should be worn: *Its force [is active] when one carries it in his hand or in the left wing (?) of his garment* → "[...] la deit l'um porter el senestre braz" (You have to wear it on the left arm.) (FP I).

The source of Berakhyah's assertion that the stone protects from reptiles could not be retrieved.

2. *acates*

Berakhyah's description of the *acates* goes to a large extent back to the First French Version of Marbode[74] (FF), especially concerning the places where the stone is found and the description of its physical aspect.

[73] *First Anglo-Norman Prose Lapidary* and *Second Anglo-Norman Prose Lapidary*, both ed. Studer & Evans (1924).

[74] *The First French Version of Marbode's Lapidary*, ed. Studer & Evans (1924).

Acates: it is so called after a river from which it is won, and which is in the land of Sicily → "Acátes est céste apelée / Por une eve ú el ést truvée, / Ke apelée est par cest num. / En Sezíle la trove l'um" (This one is called *acátes* after a river where it is found; [the stone] is called after its name. It is found in Sicily.) (FF 89–92); *It is black [...]. Embedded in it are various kinds of shapes, which are not man-made* → "Neire est e á plesurs figúres / En li formées de natures" (It is black and has various forms, in natural shapes.) (FF 93–94); *In the land of Crete the coral stone is found, which resembles it [lit. them], except that it has hues similar to gold* → "Une altre acate rest trovée / En Crete, dum est apportée; / De coral porte la figure: / Grains d'or í a peinz de nature" (Another agate is found in Crete, from where it is brought; it has the form of coral: it has naturally golden grains painted in it.) (FF 99–102).

The power of the *acates* to satiate the thirsty soul is also stated in the FF (109–110), whereas the supposed faculty of protecting against reptiles is taken from the Alphabetical Lapidary[75] (AL): "Ke, qui sur sei la porterat, / De puinture le defendrat / De scorpion et de serpent [...]" (The one who will carry it will be protected against the stings of scorpions and bites of snakes.) (AL 37–39).

For some issues—especially those mentioned at the end of the passage—, namely that it provides light to dim eyes, emanates an odor when burnt, and comforts grief, no source could be found.

3. *alectoire*

Almost all the information given for the *alectoire* is taken from the Cambridge Version of Marbode. To start with the way of obtaining the stone: *Three years after the castration of the cock this stone, which is named after it, grows close to its stomach* → "Quant li chapuns est chapunez / Et il as ses treis anz passez, / Naist ceste pire enz la ventraille" (When the capon is castrated and when it is three years old, this stone grows in the stomach.) (CL 107–109); *[...] it is removed from the cock at the right time, which is seven years after the castration, [at which time] it is full-grown. The largest one resembles a bean which is called "feve". Its aspect is white, like crystal [...]* → "Quant li chapuns avra set anz, / La pire ert parcreüe et granz. / D'une feve ad la grossecce / E del cristal ad la blanchesse"

[75] *The Alphabetical Lapidary*, ed. Studer & Evans (1924).

(When the capon will be seven years old, the stone will be full-grown and big. It has the size of a bean and the white colour of crystal.) (CL 111–114).

The information concerning its virtues—the fact that its owner defeats enemies in war, that it prevents from thirst, and that it renders pleasing—, goes back to the CL (cf. CL 115–124), too. The last sentence of Berakhyah seems to be a translation of the CL: *Ladies wear it to please men, and it is extremely powerful when one carries it in his mouth* → "A la dame ad grant valur / Ki voelt pleisir a sun seignur. / Ki ces vertuz voudra sentir / En sa buche l'estoet tenir" (It has a great value for the lady who wants to please her husband. Whoever wants to feel its powers has to hold it in his mouth.) (CL 125–128).

We did not find a source for the other virtues, e.g., increasing wealth, arousing sexual desire and being beneficial for women in hard labour.

4. *esmeralde*

The Cambridge Version of Marbode shows for the major part of Berakhyah's description a nearly literal parallel: *This stone exists in twelve varieties of colour* → "Puet l'en truver duze manieres" (You can find twelve varieties) (CL 192); *Some can be found in copper mines […]* → "Encor en est altre manire / Que l'en trove en la minire / La u l'araim solent trover" (There is another variety, which you can find in the mines where usually copper is found.) (CL 197–199); *The choicest ones come from the land of Scythia [?]. The inhabitants of the island called "Gryphons" go and surround an island whose inhabitants is a nation called "Arismapi," who have neither a head nor a brain, but have one eye on the chest. Those called "Gryphons" wait in ambush for the people called "Arismapi" when they collect the stones from the profound depths [of the sea], and [rob] them of their stones* → "De Cithie vienent les meillurs, / […] / Çoe est uns illes tut ruunt, / Li griffun herbergié i sunt; / En cele terre ad une gent / Kis asaillent mult suvent: / Arimaspi sunt apelé, / Il n'unt qu'un oil en verité. / Cil n'unt ne teste ne cerviz, / Mais k'un sul uil en mi le piz; / Icestes pieres quant voleient, / Par engin tolir lur soleient" (The best ones come from Scythia; this is a completely round island, where the "Gryphons" live; in this land there is a nation that is very often attacked by them: These people are called "Arimaspi", and actually, they have only one eye. They have neither a head nor a brain, but only one eye in the middle of the chest; when they want to have those stones, they usually rob them by ambush.) (CL 205–216).

This stone, when good, the sun does not warm, and it shines even in the dark → "Soleil ne mue sa manire, / ne umbre, [...]" (Neither the sun troubles its nature, nor darkness.) (CL 219); *If you find in it a concavity you can see your face in it, just as you see your reflected image in the water* → "En cele ki ad caveüre / Ki bien esguarde par desure / Puet l'en veeir tut ensement / Cum en claire eue sun umbre gent." (Whoever looks closely at the one that has a concavity, can see himself entirely, just as the reflected image in clear water) (CL 221–224); *A king called "Nero" had such a stone, a very large one, at which he used to look when his army was fighting and he would [fore]see the victory* → "Neiruns en ot un mireür, / Ki fud de Rume empereür; / Quant voleit veeir les melleies / Que cil feseient de espeies, / En sa piere reguardeit / Et les melleies bien veeit" (Nero, who was emperor of Rome, had a mirror of it; when he wanted to see his soldiers, what they did with their swords, he looked in [the mirror of] this stone and could clearly see his soldiers.) (CL 225–230); *He who wears it around his neck will speak well, and will respond to everyone as he sees fit.* → "Ki a sun col la portereit / Respondre a tute gent purreit" (Whoever wears it around his neck will be able to respond to everyone) (CL 237–238); *In times of thunder it has the capacity to take away fear* → "Cuntre tempestre ad grant valur" (It is helpful against thunderstorms) (CL 242); *He who wants to preserve the colour of this stone, should [wash] it in wine and then rub it with verdant olive oil* → "Ki sa verdur velt bien guarder, / En vin la cuvient a laver / E puis uindre d'olie d'olive, / Ki si seit verz cum une cive" (He who wants to preserve its green colour, should wash it in wine and then rub it with olive oil, which should be green like an onion) (CL 243–246).

Indeed, the information that the stone is good against epilepsy can be found in the Third Prose Version of Marbode[76] (TP): *Someone suffering from a hot disease [fever] or from epilepsy should wear it around his neck* → "Et qui la porte a sen col, si deffent l'oume de fievres et de goute kaiwe" (And he who wears it around his neck, it protects him against fever and epilepsy.) (TP V).

5. *onicle*

For the *onicle*, we could find parallels in the Cambridge Version of Marbode and the First French Version of Marbode as well as in the Alphabetical Lapidary. The (negative) virtues of the stone described by

[76] *Third Anglo-Norman Prose Lapidary*, ed. Studer & Evans (1924).

Berakhyah—inducing bad dreams, arousing strife and causing spitting out saliva—are taken from the CL (267–274). For the practice with the lamb's skin for preventing a child's crying, no source could be found.

The information that the harmful faculties of the *onicle* are neutralized by the *sard* (cf. entries no. 64, 65 and 67) is taken from the FF (288–290).

The description of the place where the *onicle* can be found and of its physical aspect has the closest parallel in the AL (1549–1552).

6. *etite*

Once more, the Cambridge Version of Marbode corresponds with Berakhyah more than any other lapidary; the order of the issues agrees as well (in contrast to other medieval French Marbode versions). For the most conspicuous parallels with the CL, cf. the following passages:

It can be found in the great sea that is called "Ocean" or in the kingdom of Persia, in eagles' nests. For the eagle carries it into the nest of its fledglings because the power of this stone protects them so that they do not go outside the nest and fall to the ground → "En la mer de Occeanum / Ou en Perse la regiun / Ou el ni d'aigle la querrez; / En un des trois la troverez. / Kar l'aigle en aliene terre / Va ceste pierre mult loinz querre, / Pui en son ni la va poser / Pur toz ses oiselez garder: / Ja pur tant cum el ni sera / Uns des oisaus jus ne charra" (You look for it in the Ocean or in the kingdom of Persia or in the eagle's nest; in one of those three you will find it. For the eagle goes to foreign countries and looks for this stone far away; then it will put it in its nest for protecting all its fledgling: as soon as it is in the nest, no bird will fall on the ground) (CL 623–632); *This stone is doubtless powerful, for in a house in which it is a woman will not miscarry* → "E a la femme est mult vaillant / Ki va mel de son enfant: / En la maison ou el sera / Ja femme n'i avortera" (And it is very helpful for a woman who has a difficult pregnancy: in a house in which it will be a woman will never miscarry) (CL 637–640).

If someone doubts whether or not a person hates him and he fears that that person might poison his beverage or food, and he wants to test whether this person hates him, he should invite him to eat with him from the same bowl of good food and place this stone in the bowl without that person's knowledge. Then, if that person hates him and intends to harm him he will not be able to eat anything from that food. But once he removes the stone, he will eat immediately → "Et se vos avez suspeçon / Que nus vos voille se bien non, / Que il vos voille envenimer / Ou entochier ou afoler, / Se vos esprover le volez, / Al disner le me semonez / E puis pernez une escuele / Qui mult soit bone et bele, / De quel mangier ke vos vodroiz, / La piere dedenz poseroiz: / Se culpable est, n'en gustera, / Ja si grant peine n'i metra; / La piere ostez, tot erralment / En mangera hastivement" (And if you doubt whether anyone means it well with you or not, whether he wants to envenom, poison and harm you, invite him to dinner, and then take a very precious and beautiful bowl, from which you want to eat and place the stone in it: If the person is guilty, he will not eat from it, as much as he tries it; remove the stone, quasi accidentally, and he will eat from it immediately) (CL 649–662); *There were twins in the land of Arabia who wore that stone [...]* → "Dui jomel soloient porter / La piere dont m'oez parler: / Nomé estoient a cel jor / Li uns Pollux, l'autre Castor" (Twins used to wear the stone of which you hear me speak: they were called at that time the one Pollux, the other Castor) (CL 663–666).

7. *heliotrope*

All the information concerning the *heliotrope* mentioned by Berakhyah also features in the Cambridge Version of Marbode; for some issues, we have the impression of a literal translation of this source.

Its lustre tends somewhat towards the green of the emerald stone → "De esmeraude a la color" (It has the colour of the emerald.) (CL 769); *If someone puts it in a water vessel, it changes the sunlight, so that it becomes red like blood* → "Ki la metra en un vaissel / Plain de clere eue, bon et bel, / La clareté mue del soleil, / Com sanc le fait estre vermeil, [...]" (He who puts it well in a vessel full of clear water, it changes the brightness of the sun; it makes it red like blood.) (CL 741–744); *The one who wears it knows future things and can foretell them* → "E ki ensemble o lui avra, / Mult sovent en devinera; / Des choses qui sunt a venir" (And he who will have it with him, will often know things that will happen in the future.) (CL 751–753); *He who wears it on one of his fingers will attract glory and honor and health on himself as long as he wears it* → "Ki ceste avra enz en son dei, / Los e bonté avra en soi, / Sains et halegres lungement / Iert trek'a son definement" (He who wears it on his finger will attract honor and merit, he will be healthy and save until his death.) (CL 755–757); *It stops bleeding [...]* → "Par ceste piere estanchera nes plaie ki seignera" (This stone will even stop a bleeding wound.) (CL 759); *There is a homonymous herb [such that] the one who knows [the appropriate] incantation over both of them can take as he pleases wealth from its owner.*

→ "Ki l'erbe avroit ki a sun non / E ambedeus savroit charmer, / Devant vos toz porroit aler / E prendre quanke il voldroit" (He who has the herb that has its name and who knows to enchant both, can walk in front of you all and take as much as he wants.) (CL 764–767); *[These stones] can be found in the land of Africa, Ethiopia and Cyprus* → "En Aufrike et en Ethyope / Trove l'en eliotrope; / Et Cypre [...]." (You can find the heliotrope in Africa and in Ethiopia; and [in] Cyprus ...) (CL 771–773).

8. *abeste*

The source of Berakhyah could not be identified. The lapidary tradition of Pliny—Isidore—Marbode gives other informations concerning the virtues of this stone. Yet the fact that the *abeste* can be found in the land of Arcadia is also mentioned in the medieval Marbode versions, e.g., in the First French Version (FF 673–674).

9. *ematite*

For the *ematite*, Berakhyah took the information from the Cambridge Version of Marbode. We can identify this lapidarium clearly as the source, since this version has, firstly, nearly all the issues mentioned by Berakhyah and, secondly, it is the only one to compare the colour of the hemathite to rusty iron (in contrast to the other Marbode versions, which compare it to blood): *The Arabs (= Greeks?) named it thus in their language because it somewhat resembles rust of iron* → "En gregeis est apelee / Ematite et nomee / Pur çoe k'un poi trait en rufur: / Com roil de fer est sa color" (The Greeks named it *ematite*, and it is called like this because it tends a little bit toward red: like rusty iron is its colour.) (CL 829–832). The CL is, moreover, the only text to mention the *collyrium* (an eye-salve) in the connection with the faculty of the stone of healing eye diseases: *It heals eye illness: when one touches one's eyelids with it, and having his eyes red like mutton, he should take some of its powder together with egg white, mix them well and put it on the eyes, and he will be healed. [...] Physicians who have some of this stone make from it a collyrium (eye-salve)* → "Ki malvais mal es eils avra / De ceste piere i tochera / As palpires tot entor: / Mult tost en chace la dolor. / Ki a muez ielz, com char de boef / Sa puldre ovec album de l'oef / Tres bien ensemble triblera, / Sor l'oil le mete, si garra; / Et li fisicien ki l'ont / Collirie merveillus en funt" (He who has a bad illness in his eyes, should touch them with this stone, [that is] at the eyelids all around: very soon [the stone] alleviates the pain. He who has eyes red like ox flesh, should thoroughly [mix] its powder with egg white and put it on the eye, thus, he will recover. And the physicians who have it make from it a marvellous collyrium.) (CL 843–848) (CL 847–848).

The information that the stone heals blood spitting, excessive menstruations, and diarrhea goes also back to the CL (cf. CL 849–860), as well as the reference to its efficacy against dead flesh and the bites of reptiles (cf. CL 857–864) and of the places where the *ematis* is found (cf. CL 872–874).

10. *abeste*

In contrast to the issues featuring in entry no. 8 (also *abeste*), where the source could not be found, the information about the virtues of this stone can be identified as taken from the Cambridge Version: *Its luminousness is like that of of pure (unadulterated) iron. This stone is found in Arabia, and is highly marvelous. He who kindles it, will dispose of an eternal flame that he will not be able to extinguish. He who has this stone does not need even a single candle* → "En Archadie a une piere, / Merveilluse est sa manire: / Ki une foiz l'alumeroit, / Jamais par home n'estandroit. / Mult par est bone sa nature; / Sa lumire toz tens dure. / A povre home avroit mestier / Pur sa lumire a esparnier. / De cler fer a ceste color, / Merveluse est sa vigor" (In Arcadia there is a stone, and it has a marvelous nature: once kindled, nobody could ever extinguish it. Its nature is very good; its light lasts always. It would render a good service for a poor man by saving [on the costs of] lighting. This one has the colour of brilliant iron, its nature is marvelous.) (CL 875–884).

11. *exacontalithos*

The Cambridge Version of Marbode has—as the only O. Fr. Marbode descendant—all the issues featuring in Berakhyah and can thus clearly be identified as the source of the information about this stone (although the CL has the O. Fr. term *exacontalite* and not the Gr.-Lat. form). See, e.g., the following passage:

Although small [in size], it is yet very large in vigor, for all the powers found in the other stones are present in this stone → "Mult est petite en corsage, / De vertuz a bien grant barnage: / Les vertus k'altres pieres ont / En ceste sule totes sunt" (It has a very small size, yet its virtues have a high quality: the powers of all the other stones are all of them present in this single stone.) (CL 971–974).

12. *orite*

Once again, we find all issues concerning the *orite* featuring in Berakhyah in the Cambridge Version of Marbode, so that we can determine the CL as the source here. See, e.g., the following very close parallel: *Its power is to heal wounds inflicted by wild animals. If someone pulverizes it with rose water and drinks it, will heal his wounds* → "Les plaies garist sainement / Que males bestes font a gent; Kil trible ovoec l'oile rosé, / N'en avra mont quant iert sané" (It heals the wounds that wild animals inflict upon men; he who pulverizes it with rose oil won't have it [i.e. the wound] any longer, and he will be healed.) (CL 1079–1082).

13. *enidre*

Since the Cambridge Version is the only O. Fr. Marbode text to treat the *enidre* and all issues mentioned by Berakhyah (the fact of exuding water and its hardness) figure there, the CL is clearly his source for this stone. Cf., e.g.: *For just as abundant water gushes out of a spring [without exhausting it], so also water gushes out of it* → "Tot ensement com de funtaine / En ist bele eue clere et saine" (Just like from a spring, so also clear and healthy water gushes out of it.) (CL 1135–1136).

14. *ametiste*

For this stone, we could find the closest parallels in the First French Version of Marbode and the Second Prose Lapidary. In the FF, we have the comparison of its colour to the violet (cf. FF 383) and to the red wine mixed with water (cf. FF 386) as well as the reference to five varieties (cf. FF 394), the easiness of quarrying it (cf. FF 388), and its faculty of protecting from getting drunk (cf. FF 389). For the last virtue, cf. the parallel to the SP: *It [...] is useful [...] for skillful hunters, fieldmen, for they will be successful in their hunting* → "Seurement poet chacar ki l'ad, kar ele est de si grant vertu ke les bestes sauvages venent a celuy ky la porte." (He who has it can hunt securely, because it has such a great power that the wild animals come to the one who wears it.) (SP XIV).

The etymological explication of the term—the name derives from the Gr. αἷμα, i.e., 'blood', because of its resemblance to blood—is also given in Latin Marbode (cf. Marb. Red. lap. XXXII, 1), but does not feature in the O. Fr. versions.

15. *alemandine*

Berakhyah's source for this stone could not be identified with certainty. We find parallels to the O. Fr. Marbode versions concerning the content, but in view of the wording, none of them seems to have served as a direct source. See, e.g., the following tradition with a textual parallel to the Cambridge Version of Marbode: *We do not know all of its virtues [...]* → "Ki de lui tienent jugement, / Al jugier faillent mult sovent" (Those who know about it are often wrong in their appraisal.) (CL 571–572) and to the Alphabetical Lapidary: *If you put it in cold water, it will warm up* → "E qui lungement la i larra, / Senz autre fu l'ewe buildra" (And if you will leave it for a long time in there [i.e., in the water], the water will boil without any other fire.) (AL 193–194).

16. *yenia*

For this stone, the Cambridge Version of Marbode clearly seems to be the source of Berakhyah, since many issues feature only in this text.

We do not know where [this stone] comes from. Many say that it is found in the eyes of an animal called 'hyena'. For from the eye of this animal they take the pupil → "Ne sai en laquel region / A une beste, hyene a non. / De ses oilz prent l'en les pruneles" (I don't know in which region, there is a wild animal called *hyene*. From its eyes they take the pupil.) (CL 1103–1105); *He who wears this stone can foretell the future as he wishes, if he washes this stone and puts it under his tongue* → "Ki ceste piere portera, / Une dete en soi avra: / Devinera a son plaisir / Les choses ki sunt a venir; / La bouche li covient laver / Et laienz la piere poser / Desoz la langue netement." (He who wears this stone, has a gift: He will be able to foretell future things as he wishes; he should wash his mouth and put the stone in there, just under the tongue.) (CL 1109–1115).

17. *iris*

The Cambridge Version of Marbode is the only text that lists nearly all issues we find in Berakhyah (although not in the same order), so that we can say with the utmost probability that the CL is once more the basis of Berakhyah's text:

This stone hails from the Red Sea → "[...] il vient de la Ruge Mer" (It hails from the Red Sea.) (CL 1150); *Its colour is like that of the crystal* → "Cristalline est sa color" (CL 1153); *The Arabs love [this stone] [...]* → "Cil d'Arabye le vont quere" (Those from Arabia get it.) (CL 1151); *It always has six sides (hexagonal)* → "Sis angles a sa forme entor" (Its outer form has six sides.) (CL 1154); *If one holds it up in a house against the rising sun, [i.e. with the sun] shining opposite to him, he will see on the walls of the house a few colours, like those of the rainbow in the sky* → "Ki en la maison le tendra / El rai ki del soleil vendra, / L'arc el ciel porra veoir / En sa maisiere aparoir, / E totes ses colors numbrer" (He who will hold it up in a house against the rays that come from the sun, will be able to see the rainbow appear in his house and list all its colours.) (CL 1155–1159).

18. *androdragma*

Here again, the Cambridge Version of Marbode must be the source of Berakhyah. Firstly, we can find all issues there, and secondly, the literal parallels are very close:

You find it in the sand on the seashore → "Anthrodragme solt l'en trover / El sablon de la Ruge Mer" (You usually find the *anthrodragme* in the sandy beach of the Red Sea.) (CL 1161–1162); *Its appearance is like that of refined silver. It is as hard as the diamant* → "Color a d'argent cler luisant. Dure est com piere d'aïmant" (It has the colour of bright and shining silver. It is as hard as the diamant stone.) (CL 1165–1166); *It is good to calm wrath and anger* → "Çoe dient ki sor li l'avra / Quant iriez iert, en pais serra" (They say that he who wears it, if he becomes angry, he will be soothed.) (CL 1169–1170).

19. *optallie*

The information for this stone is derived once again from the Cambridge Version of Marbode. No other text source has such close parallels:

This stone has the power to heal the eye [...] → "Optallies totes dolors / Des oilz trait hors par ses vigors" (*Optallies* relieves by its virtues every pain of the eyes.) (CL 1171–1172); *Thieves wear it while they search houses, for it affords them light in the dark and they see all that is in the house. But those who are in the house do not see or notice them. The [thieves] thus take whatever they wish* → "Çoe est la piere as larrons / Quant vont embler, brisier maisons; / Kar cil ki avoec lui l'avra, / Mult clerement toz tens vera; / Cil ki de juste li seront, / Des oilz dunt voient nel verront: / Si porra tot a son talent / Prendre l'avoir, l'or et l'argent" (Thus, the stone is [useful] for thieves when they go to break into houses;

for he who carries it will always see clearly; those who will be next to him will not see him with their eyes: Thus, he will be able to take the goods, gold and silver as he wishes.) (CL 1173–1180).

20. *absite*

Since we find the closest parallels in the Cambridge Version, this Marbode version might be Berakhyah's direct source. All the traditions mentioned by Berakhyah also feature in the CL:

It is black with red [veins] → "Neire piere est absite. / Sa maniere est en livre escrite: / De roges veines est venee" (*Absite* is a black stone. Its nature is described in the books: It is brindled with red veins.) (CL 1245–1247); *It weighs more than anything of the same size* → "Plus poise asez, quant est pesee, / Qu'ele meïsme n'a de gros, / Ou fer ou fust ou piere ou os" (When it is weighed it [has] by far more weight than things that have the same size, [e.g.,] iron, wood, stone or bone.) (CL 1248–1250); *If someone heats it in fire a single time, it remains hot during all seven days* → "Qui une foiz l'eschauferoit / Al feu, set jorz chaude seroit." (If someone heats it in the fire one time, it will remain hot for seven days.) (CL 1251–1252).

21. *electrum*

Marbode and his Angl.-Nor. literary descendants are not the source of Berakhyah here. In the Angl.-Nor. lapidaries, the *electrum* does not feature seperately as a single stone, but is described in those passages that treat the *lyncurium* as a stone that resembles it, cf., e.g.: "Li boens auctors Theofrastés / Dit k'electre semble pres: / C'est une gemme clere et bele, / Toz tens est en clarté novele. / Une force ont, une valor, / De pailes traire par vigor" (The trustworthy author Theophrastus says that the *electre* ressembles it [i.e., the *lyncurium*] a little bit in attracting straw by its force.) (CL 611–616).

We could rather find direct correspondences to Latin sources, namely Pliny, Isidore and Albertus Magnus: the comparison of the colour to wax could be retrieved in Pliny: *It looks like wax* → "Candidum atque cerei coloris quod vocaretur electrum" (Plin. nat. XXXVII, 33); its transparency is mentioned in Albertus Magnus: *Its opaqueness [i.e. transparence] is the same as that of [rock-]crystal* → "Sometimes it is found as transparent as glass" (Albert. M. miner.[77] II, 2, 17).

[77] Albertus Magnus, *Book of Minerals (Mineralia)*, transl. Wyckoff (1976).

In Pliny, Isidore and Albertus Magnus, we also find the observation that the *electrum* burns (Plin. nat. XXXVII, 43; Isid. nat. orig.[78] XVI, 8, 6; Albert. M. loc. cit.) and that it attracts straw (Plin. nat. XXXVII, 48; Isid. nat. orig. XVI, 8, 7; Albert. M. loc. cit.).

22. *optallius*

For the *optallius*, we could find the closest parallels in Isidore's description of the *opalus*:

This stone has dissimilar colours → "Opalus distinctus diversarum colore gemmarum. [...], et cuncta pariter sub quadam varietate lucentia" (Isid. nat. orig. XVI, 12, 3); *Its name is that of a city in the land of India* → "Nomen habet ex patria; sola enim eum parturit India" (loc. cit.); *Some of it are luminous like a flame, and thereby resemble the carbuncle, while the vigor of its luminousness is similar to that of the aematite. It also has a green [tint] like the emerald* → "Est enim in eo carbunculi tenuior ignis, amethysti fulgens purpura, smaragdi nitens viriditas" (loc. cit.).

The remaining mentioned virtues (curing eye diseases, rendering invisible) do neither figure in Isidore nor in Pliny nor in Albertus Magnus, but can be retrieved in Lat. and Angl.-Nor. Marbode (cf. entry no. 19), originally taken from Damigeron: *He who wears it will be cured from eye-ache. If he is a thief, he will not be caught while he still wears it* → "Optallius[79] lapis circa oculos efficax est; nam qui gerit eum, numquam oculis laborabit. Aptus est autem et furibus, ut non teneantur" (Damig. lap.[80] XXIV).

For the faculty of the *optallius* of breaking iron chains, no source could be retrieved.

323. **ancotre*

This stone could not be identified (cf. section 2). We might think of a relation to the *acintitota*, which appears in the Lat. abridgement[81] of the Alphabetical Lapidary. This Lat. text is a retranslation from the O. Fr.

[78] Isidorus Hispalensis, *Etymologiarum sive originum libri XX (De natura rerum origines)*, ed. Lindsay (1911).

[79] It is remarkable that Damigeron has a nearly corresponding form to Berakhyah (in contrast to *opalus* in the other Lat. texts)—may we take this as an index of being the source?

[80] Damigeron, *De lapidibus*, ed. Abel (1881).

[81] Ed. Meyer (1909).

poem. In spite of the fact that this text originates from Italy and that the spelling of our stone name differs seriously from *acintitota*, we find considerable parallels concerning the content: For the first issue, cf. the Lat. abridgement: *It somewhat resembles [rock-]crystal but it is not as transparent* → "Acintitota est lapis similis cristallo" (Meyer 1909:549); also cf. Isidore: "Iacinthizonta [...]. Quidam autem eorum crystalli similes" (Isid. nat. orig. XVI, 9, 3).

For the other virtues, no source could be found.

24. **asistos*

No sources were found for this stone, which could not be identified (cf. section 2).

25. *ambra*

No sources could be found for this stone, which is missing in Marbode.

26. *asterites*

This stone is not present in the Marbode tradition, but for a close parallel, cf. Isidore: *Light is enclosed in it, seemingly moving within it like the light of a star. It turns the sun's brilliance into white* → "Asterites candida est, inclusam lucem continens veluti stellam intus ambulantem, redditque solis candicantes radios" (Isid. nat. orig. XVI, 10, 3).

27. *amiantus*

The consulted texts give other information about the *amiantus* than Berakhyah. The properties mentioned in our text rather correspond to those of the hemathite (cf. entry no. 9), so that we can not identify the source here.

28. *beril*

The traditions about the *beril* are taken from the Cambridge Version of Marbode and from the Alphabetical Lapidary. We find there similar descriptions of its physical aspect, i.e., the comparison to sea water (cf. CL 314) and its suitability of being cutted with six facets (cf. CL 309–

310). For the virtues of the *beril*, the CL mentions also the faculties of drawing a man's love to his wife (cf. CL 316), of increasing honor (cf. CL 319–320) and of burning the hand when the stone is held in it (cf. CL 322).

Its virtue of healing eye-ache and pain in the liver goes also back to the CL: *To cure the redness of the eye, one should leave it in water for one night and rinse his eyes with that water* → "E ki de l'eue u ele gist / Met en ses oelz, de mal guarist" (And he who rinses his eyes with the water in which it had been put will be cured of the pain.) (CL 323–324); *If someone daily drinks water in which it was immersed it will [...] cure him from pain in the liver* → "E ki l'eue use chascun jur, / Del feie li tot la dulur" (And he who uses the water every day will be cured of liver pain.) (CL 325–326).

The tradition that the *beril* is able to ignite dry things when hold against the sun is, indeed, borrowed from the AL: *If you hold this stone against the sun, you can ignite a piece of cloth or* ⟨...⟩ → "Le rai del soleil trait a sei. / E li rais est est d'itel nature / Qu'il la tresperce sanz fraiture, / E si est chaut de altre part, / Que il esprent e bruille e art / Estupes, tundre, drapelez, / Seches choses et estramés" (It attracts the sunbeam, and the sunbeam has the property to penetrate it [i.e. the stone] without breaking it. And it [i.e. the sunbeam] is so hot on the other side that it burns and ignites and scorches tow, tinder, clothes, dry things and straw.) (AL 226–232).

Its powers of curing gout and of protecting from drowning could not be retrieved in the consulted sources.

29. *grisolite*

For this stone, several Angl.-Nor. Marbode versions, i.e. the First French Version (FF), the Cambridge Version (CL), the First Prose Lapidary (FP), and the Alphabetical Lapidary (AL), have to be considered. For the single issues, cf. the following close parallels:

Its colour is like that of the sea, and within it there is what looks like a gold granule → "Si a semblant d'eue de mer. / Enz a un grain d'or el milou" (It is similar to sea water. It has a gold granule in the middle of it.) (FF 298–299); *When it is set in pure gold, its hue is like that of a burning coal. When it is in the shade you can distinguish in it a green colour* → "Quant ele siet en fin or cler, / Cum carbun deit restenceler. / Quant vient en umbre, sa culur / Trait un petit envers verdur" (When it is in fine and bright gold, it sparkles like coal. When it comes into the shadow, it becomes a little bit green.) (CL 293–296); *The one who wears it need not fear wild animals*

→ "Ele est mult bone a porter sur sei cuntre naturals pours." (It is very good to wear it against fears caused by nature [i.e., animals].) (FP VII); *If you find it pierced, pass a hair from the tail of an ass through the hole: it is then beneficial for madmen, to bring them back to their mind* → "[...] ki l'ad perciede, et dunches met parmi le pertus seie de asne, si em pot l'um dechacier les diables" (He who has a pierced [stone], pass an hair of an ass through the hole, then you can chase away the evil spirits.) (FP VII); *He who suffers from nightmares should wear it [encased] in a ring of tin or lead on his left hand* → "Ker ceste pere ad valur / Encuntre nocturnel poür." (Because this stone has the power against nightmares.) (AL 541–542).

For the other issues, no sources could be found.

30. *grisopras*

The comparison of the stone's colour to leek soup is present in nearly all Angl.-Nor. Marbode versions. Its beneficial effect against epilepsy is only present in the Apocalyptical Lapidary:[82] *It is beneficial for an epileptic* → "Fevre ne gute nen avrad" (He will neither have fever nor epilepsy.) (AP 213).

The textual origin of the stone's power of being beneficial against arthritis could not be found.

31. *crisopacion*

Just as here, in the *Ko'aḥ ha-Avanim*, this stone figures twice in Marbode (Marb. Red. lap. XV—*crisoprassus* and LX—*crisopacion*). Riddle assumes that Marbode mistakenly "confused the variant descriptions as being for two stones" (Riddle 1977:90–91). This double occurrence is adopted in the First French Version and the Cambridge Version of Marbode, from where it is taken by Berakhyah. The CL has the closer textual parallel concerning the following issue: *In the dark you can perceive its luminousness, but during the day you do not discern luminousness in it* → "Par nuit luist mult clere la piere, / De jorz pert tote sa lumire; / La nuit luist, palist le jor" (By night, the stone shines very bright, during the day, it looses its light; it shines by night, during the day it turns pale.) (CL 1345–1347).

No source could be retrieved for the faculties of alleviating thirst and comforting the mind.

---

[82] *The Apocalyptic Lapidary*, ed. Studer & Evans (1924).

32. *gagatromé*

The textual parallels of Berakhyah's text to the Cambridge Version of Marbode are obvious: *By its spots it resembles the hair [pelt] of a lamb* → "[…] a pel de chevrel est semblant" (It resembles the hair of a goat.) (CL 694); *The one who wears it will be dreaded by his enemies. An ancient king used to wear it in battle, and was victorious as long as he wore it; one day he forgot [to wear] it and was killed* → "Cil ki sor lui la portera, / Trestoz ses enemis vaintra, […]. / Par ceste piere Alcidés / Maint peril veinqui; aprés, / Un jor la lassa, çoe m'est vis; / Ocis fu de ses enemis" (He who wears it will defeat all his enemies. With the aid of this stone, Hercules averted many dangers; but then, one day he forgot it, as it seems to me, and he was killed by his enemies.) (CL 695–702).

33. *galactites*

For the *galactites*, the Cambridge Version of Marbode is again clearly Berakhyah's source. We find there the comparison of the stone's colour to ashes (cf. CL 1042), its faculty of increasing the milk production (cf. CL 1043–1045), and the comparison of its taste to milk (cf. CL 1075–1076).

Close textual parallels can be found for the procedure to be followed when the shepherd wants his herd to produce more milk and for unproblematic parturitions of the ewes: *If someone weaves a thread from the wool of an ewe, perforates this stone, and hangs it around her neck with this thread, she will have plenty of milk. If she [the ewe] has a difficult parturition, he [the shepherd] should attach the stone to her belly, fastened with the mentioned thread* → "Un poi de laine ki prendroit / De la berbiz ki grief seroit / Et un fort fil puis enfilast / Et ceste piere partusast / Et le fil par mi meïst / Et a son col puis la pendist, / Del lait avreit tot ensement / […]. / Ki vad mel de son enfant, / Mais sor son ventre soit liee / Al fil dont parol atachiee" (Someone who takes a little bit of wool of an ewe that is pregnant and then weaves a strong thread and perforates the stone and puts the thread through the middle and then hangs it around her neck, will soon have plenty of milk. If she has a difficult parturition, it should be bound on her belly and attached with the mentioned thread.) (CL 1047–1058); *If someone wants his herd to [produce] much milk, he should wash this stone with pure water and salt and besprinkle his herd with it ere the sun rises: he will then have plenty of milk* → "Ki de ses berbiz voelt foison / De lait aver en sa maison, / […] / E puis la piere triblera / A l'eue clere et al sel: / [...]; / Einz ke li soleilz soit levez / Soit li berzilz bein arosez: / Li lait forment habundera" (He who wants to have an abundance of milk in his home should grind [the stone], then wash it with pure water and with salt; before the sun has risen, the herd should be well besprinkled: he will have milk abundantly.) (CL 1059–1067).

The warning that, carried in the mouth, the stone confuses the mind, is also present in the CL (cf. CL 1073–1074).

34. **galictotea*

No source could be found for this stone, nor could it be identified (cf. section 2).

35. *gelazias*

Both the Cambridge Version and the Alphabetical Lapidary could be the source for Berakhyah's description of the *gelazias*. The AL gives the variant *galacias* (AL 1161), which is, indeed, closer to the Hebrew spelling (in contrast to *gelace* in the CL 959) and could thus be regarded as the primary source: *[This stone] is entirely white, and its aspect is like that of ice. It cannot be heated by fire* → "Galacias est une pere / Cume gresille est sa manere. / [...], / Que tant est freide e engelee / Que ja pur fu n'iert eschaufee" (*Galacias* is a stone; its nature is like hail. It is so cold and frozen that it can never be heated by fire.) (AL 1161–1166).

36. *diadocode*

Since the Cambridge Version of Marbode is the only text that, firstly, lists all the traditions mentioned by Berakhyah concerning this stone, secondly, describes them in a very similar way, and, thirdly, is the only one to show the same spelling: *diadocode* (CL 1294), it is Berakhyah's most probable source:

It has the same aspect as beryl, it is pure on all its sides (facets). If someone throws it into a vessel with water, he can see as he pleases a species of demons, and they will answer whatever questions he may ask them. For there is nothing that coerces the demons to speak as well as does [this stone] → "Diadocode [...]. / Beril resemble de color, / Clere est et bele tot entor. / En l'eue ki la met gisir, / Mult poet veoir a son plaisir / Des umbres as enemis: / Diront li quanke il avront quis. / Çoe est la piere en tot le mont / Par cui deiables plus respont" (The *diadocode* resembles the beryl in its colour, it is pure and beautiful all around. He who puts it into water can see as he pleases many shadows of demons: they will tell him whatever he will have asked. For this [reason], this stone is the one through which the demons answer best of all.) (CL 1294–1302); *The scholars have therefore called it "holy", for if it is brought in contact with a corpse or with the cadaver of a bird or animal, it loses its force* → "Kar ki al cors la tocheroit, / Trestotes ses vertuz perdroit. / Iceste gemme et sa maniere / Est apelee sainte piere" (For if someone touches a cadaver with it, it will soon lose its forces. This stone and its kinds is called "holy stone".) (CL 1305–1308).

37. *dionise*

A source for this stone could not be found for all issues given by Berakhyah, but the Cambridge Version of Marbode has two textual parallels:

It is a black [stone] with red sparks. If one grinds/ pulverizes it in water, he will perceive the odor of wine → CL "Noire piere est dionise, / De gotes ruges est purprise. / Ki a l'eue la tribleroit, / Flairor de vin de li istroit" (*Dionise* is a black stone spotted with red dots. If one grinds it in water, the odor of wine will emanate from it.) (CL 1311–1314); *[...] whoever smells this stone immixed with water will not get drunk* → "Et nekedent ceste flairor / De trestoz vins tolt la vigor: / Ja nus hoem ivre ne sera / Ki ceste piere flairé a" (And in spite of this odor it neutralizes the effect of every [kind of] wine: no one will get drunk who has smelled this stone.) (CL 1315–1318).

38. *diamant*

For the *diamant*, three possible sources of Berakhyah could be identified as being mixed up: The First French Version (FF), the Third Prose Lapidary (TP) and the Cambridge Version of Marbode (CL).

For most issues, the FF has the closest parallels, e.g., for its aspect and physical properties: *Some of them have the size of a Greek bean* → "N'est grendre d'une nuiz petite" (It is not larger than a small nut.) (FF 61); *[...] and it somewhat tends towards the color of rock crystal* → "[...] el est clere cume cristal, / [...]" (It is clear like crystal.) (FF 50); *Nothing can burst it, nor is it damaged by the power of fire. However, when they want to burst it so as to make two [stones] out of one, then they take the blood of a he-goat which is still warm, boil it, and steep [the stone] in that hot blood* → "Par fer ne par fou n'iert ovree, / S'en sanc de buc chiald n'est tempree; / L'om l'i moile tan com est chialz, / [...]" (Neither by iron nor by fire can it be cut, if it is not steeped in warm gout blood; you should bathe it as long as it is warm.) (FF 53–55).

The FF also seems to be the source for the fact that magicians make use of the stone (cf. FF 73–74), that it protects from bad dreams and reptiles (cf. FF 77–79), that it calms wrath (cf. FF 80–81), and, finally, that it should be worn on the left side (cf. FF 87).

The TP (VII), indeed, is the only text that recommands to set the *diamant* in steel ("achier"; cf. the adoption of the O. Fr. word in Hebrew אֲצִ׳יר—*'aṢiYR* for *acier*, 'steel').

In the CL we find the information that the stone attracts iron—being stronger than the *magnete* (cf. CL 37–40) and that it protects from enemies (cf. CL 48).

39. *turquois*

A source for Berakhyah's description of this stone could not be identified. The *turquois* does not feature in the Marbode tradition, but is described in Albertus Magnus (Albert. M. miner. II, 2, 18). The name was given to the stone only in the Middle Ages when it was imported "from the Turks". It was probably treated by earlier writers under other names (cf. Wyckoff 1976:123).

Cf. the parallel Berakhyah—Albertus Magnus in the following passage: *[It] is opaque white, somewhat leaning toward the green. The variety which is useful for eyesight [...] has green dots* → "Turchois is a stone of a brightly shining blue colour, as if milk had penetrated the blue colour and risen to the surface through it. They say that it preserves the sight" (Albert. M. miner. loc. cit.).

40. *topace*

Originally, Pliny described the *topazos* as a green stone in two varieties: the *prasoides* and the *chrysoptreron* (cf. Plin. nat. XXXVII, 32, 107–109). Later, Isidore stressed a "golden" topaz (cf. Isid. nat. orig. XVI, 9, 10), and the name came to mean a yellow or orange stone—our topaz, but also other yellow stones like citrine quartz. In an unknown source used by Marbode (Marb. Red. lap. XIII) the stone is confused with the *hephaestites*, which was supposed to stop the boiling of water. This interpretation entered in the Angl.-Nor. Marbode traditions and was apparently also accepted by Berakhyah. Most of the other issues described by Berakhyah go back to another, unknown source.

Cf. the parallels to the Angl.-Nor. Verse Adaption of Marbode[83] (VA), which is the only source to mention the last of the following aspects: *It has two varieties* → "Dous topaces sunt trovees" (Two kinds of topaz are found.) (VA 323); *Many tried to cool boiling water with it* → "Desbullir fet l'ewe boillant" (It causes water to stop boiling.) (VA 331); *In it you see the inverted images of faces* → "Del home turne le visage / Envers, tel est le soen usage" (It inverts the faces of men; this is its habit.) (VA 337–338).

41. *jaspe*

The description of this stone has the closest parallels in the Second Prose Version of Marbode. Only the following issues can be traced back to Marbode, whereas for the other aspects, no source could be identified:

The best of all is the green [variety] → "Cele est la meudre ky est verz" (The best stone is the green one.); *It is beneficial for fever and for dropsy* → "Ele garde homme de feveres et d'ydropesie" (It preserves man from fever and dropsy.); *It is beneficial for a woman having a difficult [childbirth] and against evil spirits* → "Ele ayde a femme qui enfaunte [...]. Ele debute fantasmes nuysaunz" (It helps a woman in childbirth. It chases away evil spirits.); *It is set principally in silver* → "Sa vertu est greignur en argent k'en autre metal" (Its virtue is greater in silver than in any other metal.); *The [jasper] that is green with red drops stops bleeding and gives success* → "Ele ad gutes vermeyles [...]; et fet homme estre amé et puissaunt. [...]; ele estaunche de sanc et de meneysun" (It has red drops; it makes a man popular and successful; it stops bleeding and diarrhea.) (all SP IV).

42. *jaiet*

A combination of several Angl.-Nor. Marbode texts could be the possible source of Berakhyah for the *jaiet*. The Cambridge Version has the most parallels, e.g., concerning the stone's aspect (cf. CL 458), its beneficial virtue for a woman's menstruation flux (cf. CL 469–472) and for the ease of labour pains (cf. CL 479–482), and its power against demons (cf. CL 476). Also cf. the very close following parallels: *If someone chafes it by rubbing, it raises [i.e. attracts] the straw. If someone wishes to set it ablaze*

[83] *Anglo-Norman Verse Adaption of the 'First French Version' and Fragments of Other Verse translations of Marbode's Poem*, ed. Studer & Evans (1924).

he should wash the stone in water; it cannot then be quenched, except with olive oil → "Quant en l'eschaufe, k'il est chaut, / A soi trait les pailles en halt. / Ki velt ardoir et alumer, / De l'eue le convient laver; / D'oile d'olive, quant voldrez, / Tres bien estaindre le purrez" (If you chafe it until it is hot, it attracts straw upwards to itself. He who wants to burn it and set it ablaze, it is good to wash it in water; with olive oil, if you want, you can extinguish it very well.) (CL 459–464); *If someone fell ill with gout, which is between the skin and the flesh, he should wear [this stone] and touch [the affected spot] with it. The water in which the stone was washed strengthens loose teeth* → "Ki gute a entre char et quir / Ceste est bone a li garir. / L'eue dont l'en l'a fait laver / Les denz lochanz fait afermer" (If someone suffers from gout between skin and flesh, this [stone] is good for healing him. The water in which it was washed strengthens loose teeth.) (CL 465–468).

The power of the stone to test a woman's virginity is only mentioned by the First French Version (cf. FF 446), whereas the *jaiet's* virtue of curing an upset stomach can be found in the Third Prose Lapidary (cf. TP XVIII).

43. *gerachite*

The Cambridge Version of Marbode is clearly the source for Berakhyah's description of the *gerachite*:

It is somewhat black → "Trestote est noire sa color" (Its colour is entirely black.) (CL 779); *If someone first washes his face* [cf. Ms. A: *this stone*] *and then puts it in his mouth, he will apprehend what his companion thinks of him* → "Ki primes la lavera, / Et en sa buche la mettra, / [...] / Dire purra le pensement / C'uns autres de lui pensera" (He who washes it first and puts it in his mouth will be able to tell the thoughts that other people have about him.) (CL 781–785); *Whatever he may ask of people they will not deny him. With women he can do as he pleases* → "Ki ceste piere portera, / Ja nus ne li escundira, / [...]. / As dames iert boen sovent, / Kar ne li poent contrester / Se sulement les voelt ruver" (If someone carries this stone, nobody will deny him. He will often be [successful] with women, because they will not be able to resist, if only he wants to seduce them.) (CL 786–792); *As for testing [the stone]: [...] Even if the stone is coated with milk or honey, it will chase the flies. But when the stone is removed they return to where they were* [cf. Ms. A: *they return to attack fiercely*] → "Se vus esprover la volez, / Ki ceste piere porterez, / Oignez vos de lait et de miel, / Si fuiront com ce fust fiel / Des muches la grant compainie, / A vos ne tocheront ja mie; / Rostez la piere en sus de vos, /

Assalt mult grant et merveillus / Avrez vos mult isnelement / des muches sanz demorement: / De tutes pars vus assaldront" (If you want to test it, wear the stone and coat yourself with milk and honey; the great swarm of flies will flee as if it was gall, and they will not touch you; remove the stone from yourself, and immediately, you will have a great and terrible attack of flees without respite: they will attack you from everywhere.) (CL 793–803).

44. *gelazia*

A definite source for this stone could not be identified. However, the comparison of the stone's aspect to hail can also be found in the Cambridge Version of Marbode: *It looks like hail which is called "gresil" and is not larger than it, […]. It is always cold and you cannot heat it [even] by pure fire* → "Gresille semble ceste piere / De grossece e de manire; / […]: / Toz tens pardure en freidur, / Feu ne li puet doner chalor" (This stone resembles in its size and nature the hail; it remains always cold, fire can not heat it.) (CL 961–966).

45. **legnete*

This stone does not figure in the Marbode and the Angl.-Nor. Marbode tradition, but is described in Lat. sources, e.g., by Pliny, Damigeron and Isidore. The information about its physical aspect is taken from the Pliny / Isidore tradition (cf. Plin. nat. XXXVII, 29, 103, and Isid. nat. orig. XVI, 14, 4), as well as the fact that, heated, it attracts straw (cf. Plin. nat. loc. cit. and Isid. nat. orig. loc. cit.). The idea of the "debris of carbuncle" can also be traced back to these authors (cf. loc. cit., respectively).

For the other issues, Damigeron has the closest parallels to Berakhyah: *It is beneficial for evil spirits, and [it is beneficial] to fasten it to a man whose nose is bleeding* → "Adversus nyctalopam [id est adversus nocturnas aves, …] aptus collo est idoneus. […] in fronte ligatus fluxum sanguis stringit"; *It is beneficial for [those who speak in] riddles […]* → "Infirmos prohibet aliena loqui"; *When it is feared that a house may burn down because houses around it are on fire, one should place the stone vis-à-vis [the house], and the fire will retreat* → "Insuper si quis eum consecratum habuerit in domo quae incenditur, si casu contigerit, continuo extingitur incendium" (all Damig. lap. XXVIII).

46. *ligurie*

The colour of the *ligurie* is also described as yellow in the Verse Adaption of Marbode: "Jaune est ..." (It is yellow ...) (VA 273), whereas the Cambridge Version of Marbode seems to be the source for Berakhyah's information about the virtues of the stone: *It attracts straw to it. It cures pain and the malady of the gout [...]* → "Une force ont, une valor, / De pailes traire par vigor, / [...]. / As gotes, as autres dolors / Rent garison par ses vigors" (They have one power, one force: attracting straw by their virtue. [...] They cure gout and other pains by their virtues.) (CL 615–620).

The association of the stone with *date*, 'urine', is also present in the First Prose Lapidary: *Some call it "dațe"* → "Ligurium est piere ki creist de la date de une beste [...]" (*Ligurium* is a stone that originates from the urine of an animal.) (FP XIX).

47. *medus*

The Cambridge Version of Marbode is clearly Berakhyah's source for the *medus*. All issues figure there and are described in the same way:

Many have tried its power for someone whose eyes have been blinded through an illness. One should take this stone, mix it [i.e. its powder] with the milk of a woman who gave birth to a male child, and apply it to his eyes until his eyesight is restored → "De vertuz est bien espovee: / Li hom qui gote ne verroit, / Ki de mal avuglez seroit, / Ki un petit de ceste gemme / Destemprast od lait de femme / Ki un enfant porté eüst, / Se ke li enfes malles fust, / E ses oilz sovent en oindroit, / Aprés çoe clerement veroit" (It has been well proved with regard to its virtue: a man who can not see, who has become blind through an illness, should soak a [pulverized] piece of this stone in the milk of a woman who gave birth to a child—if the child was male—and should apply it frequently to his eyes; after that, he will see clearly.) (CL 924–932).

The reference to the healing power of the stone against gout and pain in the loins features also there (cf. CL 933–935; 943–944); the procedure of blinding one's enemy is described in the same way: *If someone wants to blind his enemy he should whet the stone on a red whetstone, [immersed] in clear water and rub some of it [i.e. the water with the stone particles] on the forehead of his enemy: he will instantly be blinded. If you let him drink from this water, he will vomit until he dies* → "Se vos vostre enemi avez, / Iceste piere triblerez / Et la cuz ruge ensement / A l'eue clere durement; /

Celui faites l'eue doner / Pur son front oindre et laver: / Si tost com il [i] tochera, / De oilz andous avoglera; / Se vos a boivre li donez, / Tant vomira k'il iert tuez" (If you have [caught] your enemy, whet this stone and a red whetstone well in clear water; give him the water, in order that he rubs and washes his forehead: as soon as he touches it, he will be blinded at both eyes; if you give it him to drink, he will vomit until he dies.) (CL 945–954).

Finally, the occurrence of two kinds of the stone (a black and a greenish-white one) can also be found in the CL (cf. CL 955–958).

48. *perle*

For the *perle*, no direct source could be found, but its supposed origin from a drop of dew is described in the First French Version of Marbode: "Li sage dient ke les mosles / Cuntre le ciel beent les gules: / La rosee del ciel receivent / E de ce les pieres cunceivent" (The sages say that the mussels open their throats against the sky: they receive the dew from the sky, and from this they produce the stones.) (FF 857–860).

49. *pantera*

Berakhyah's possible source for the description of the *pantera* might be the Second Prose Lapidary and the Cambridge Version of Marbode. The relationship with the jasper and its occurrence in many colours has a parallel in the *pantera*'s description in the SP (cf. SP XXXIII), whereas the power of the stone to provide the owner with invincibility features in the CL: *If someone wears it and looks at it before sunrise, he will be feared by everyone and will be invincible on that day* → "Ki ceste piere portera / Et chascun jor l'esgardera / Einz ke li soleilz seit levez, / De trestoz homes iert dotez; / Ja icel jor k'il la vera, / Par home veincuz ne sera" (If someone wears this stone and looks at it every day before the sun has risen, he will be feared by everyone; the day he looks at it, no one will defeat him.) (CL 1229–1234).

50. *pedoretes*

The description of this stone clearly goes back to the Cambridge Version of Marbode: *[It is] white and its luminescence is somewhat like that of gold, but at a certain distance it does not shine. The nerves of the one who wears it will not contract. Therefore, it is said that it is beneficial for the nerves* → "[U]ne gemme est pedoretés, / D'ivoire a la color pres. / Ne gete clarté, ne raïr, / Mais as nerfs a mult grant mestier; / Kar ki sor lui la portera, / Ja de nerfs ne contrara" (*Pedoretés* is a precious stone that has roughly the colour of ivory. It has no shine nor resplendence, but it is very beneficial for the nerves; for if someone wears it, his nerves will not contract.) (CL 1367–1372).

51. **paitoros*

For this unidentified stone (cf. section 2), no source could be retrieved.

52. **peritora*

The identification of this stone is unclear (cf. section 2); a source could not be found.

53. *carboncle*

Possible sources could only be found for some of the given virtues of the *charbocle*, e.g., the Cambridge Lapidary: *It burns like wood and burning coal* → "Kar ele est si reflamboiant / Cum li charbuns del feu ardant" (It is red-hot like burning coal in the fire.) (CL 589–590); *Neither darkness nor light darken its blaze* → "Nule clarté ne tenebror / Ne li puet tolir sa clarur" (Neither light nor darkness can remove its shine.) (CL 593–594).

The faculty of the stone of providing its owner with favour features also in the Verse Adaption of Marbode (cf. VA 549–550), whereas the emphasis on its blaze can be found in the First French Version of Marbode (cf. FF 520).

54. *coral*

Several Lat. and Angl.-Nor. texts could have served as a source for the description of the *coral*. Its occurrence in two different colours, its healing power against epilepsy and excessive menstrual flow, and its faculty of increasing the fruit production of herbs and trees may go back to Albertus Magnus (for all issues, cf. Albert. M. miner. II, 2, 3).

The manuscript Bodleian Digby 13, fol. 17[84] is the only text to refer to Galen: *Galen said that it cures eye ache. For toothache and a worn tooth one should rinse the stone in water and rub the teeth with that water* → "Corallus ut dicit galienus valet ad omnem dolorem oculorum et caliginem et dentium dolorem, [...] si sit bene tritus et cum cumino mixtus si dentes sint bene fricati inde et oculi loti [...]" (MJE 221).

Damigeron seems to be the source for the last two aspects, namely the faculty of the *coral* of rendering someone victorious and of protecting him from drowning, see Damigeron: "et in bello quoque et pugna maximum adiutorium est. Invictum et efficacem [...] facit gestantem eum"; "in nave hoc si habueris, multum efficacior eris: resistit autem ventis et tempestatibus et turbidinibus" (Damig. lap. VII).

The information about the protection from evil spirits may go back to an Angl.-Nor. source, the Cambridge Lapidary: "Des diables n'a poür, / Ki l'a sor soi ne nuit ne jor" (He who wears it all day and all Nicht Log, will not fear evil spirits.) (CL 563–564).

For the other issues, no source could be found.

55. *colire*

The text of the Alphabetic Lapidary corresponds well to the information given by Berakhyah, and it is the only text in the Marbode tradition to treat this stone. We can thus suppose that it is Berakhyah's source: *Its color somewhat tends towards that of a sapphire and its shining tends to that of sea water* → "El est semblable a saphire, / E si est blanche en luur, / Tel ad cumme de mer colur" (It is similar to the sapphire, and it is thus white in its shining; it has the colour of sea water.) (AL 668–670); *If someone wears it around his neck, he will not arouse the wrath and ire of the land's rulers* → "E qui iceste pere avra / E a sun col la portera, / Ja de seignur maugré n'avra" (And he who has this stone and wears it around his neck, will not incur the wrath of the land's ruler.) (AL 671–673).

56. *cornoligne*

For this stone, the Cambridge Version of Marbode seems clearly to be the source, since it mentions all issues given by Berakhyah and treats them in a similar way:

[84] In the Appendix of Evans (1922), *Magical Jewels of the Middle Ages and the Renaissance, Particularly in England* (= MJE), seven Lat. manuscripts are edited.

It is thoroughly red, and the red is very dark: it basically looks like water that has been used to wash meat → "[C]orneline est merveille oscure / Cum est [de] char la laveüre" (*Corneline* is marvellously dark like water in which meat has been washed.) (CL 573–574); *Whoever wears it on his finger or his neck will be little irascible and easy to appease* → "Qui en son col ou en son dei / La portera ensemble o soi, / [...] / [...] en ses ires met mesure" (He who wears it around his neck or on his finger, it will control his wrath.) (CL 577–580); *It stops bleeding anywhere [in the body] [...]. It is very beneficial to stop [excessive] menstrual bleeding of a woman* → "De que ke liu que li cura / Li sans, tres bien l'estanchera; / E a la femme a grant mestier / Ki de cest mal ad enconbrer" (It cures you from bleeding at every place [in the body], it stops it very well; and it is very helpful for a woman who is affected with this affliction.) (CL 581–584).

57. *cristal*

Parallels in the source texts, namely in the Cambridge version of Marbode, could only be found for the following issues:

Its whiteness is like the color of the ice → "[L]i plusor meistre de cristal / Dient que glace est ivernal, / Mult par est clere sa color, / [...]" (Most of the connoisseurs of the *cristal* say that it is hibernal ice; actually, its colour is very clear.) (CL 1016–1017); *To bring back the milk [of a breast-feeding woman]: pulverize it in honey, mix it, and let her drink it; the milk will be restored* → "As meres a mult grant mestier / Pur lor enfant bien alaiter: / Ki al miel la triblera, / Et [en] son boivre la metra, / Lait avra a son talent, / [...]" (It is very helpful for mothers to breast-feed their child: if someone pulverizes it in honey and mixes it in her beverage, she will have milk as much as she wants.) (CL 1027–1032).

58. *calcidonia*

A definite source for the *calcidonia* could not be identified; the description of its physical aspect has parallels in First French Version of Marbode: *There are three varieties [of this stone][...]* → "E de treis culurs est trovee" (And it is found in three colours). (FF 216); *[...] one is somewhat yellow; and one is median between hyacinth and beryl* → "Calcedoine est piere jalne / Entre jacint e beril meaune" (*Calcedoine* is a yellow stone, it is median between hyacinth and beryl.) (FF 207–208).

For the mentioned virtues, original Marbode comes closest, since it is the only text to mention a "pierced stone": *[...] it is beneficial to wear it on one's finger or neck. The pierced [stone] one should hang on a hair of a donkey: he who wears it will be victorious, [...]* → "Qui si pertusus digito collove geratur, / Is qui portat eum prohibetur vincere causas" (Marb. Red. lap. VI, 131–132).

For the other issues, no source could be retrieved.

59. *camahieu*

We could not retrieve a source for this stone, which does not appear in Marbode nor the Angl.-Nor. Marbode tradition—except for the Alphabetical Lapidary. However, the information the AL provides concerning this stone is different from that of Berakhyah. The text of Albertus Magnus has some parallels to the issues given by Berakhyah:

These stones mostly have projecting images → Albert. M.: "Its power is said to be due to the images and carvings found on it" (Albert. M. miner. II, 2, 9); *There are many varieties of this stone: one has white in the area [surrounding the image] and black beneath it; there is a red one; and there is a pale one* → "Kacamon is a stone that is frequently white, either wholly or in part; for it is varied in colour, and most frequently it is found mixed with onyx" (Albert. M. loc. cit.).

60. *calcofone*

The Cambridge Lapidary is probably Berakhyah's source for the information about the *calcofone*:

It is black in its entirety → "[C]alcofonie est une piere, / Trestote est noire sa maniere" (*Calcofonie* is a stone whose aspect is totally black.) (CL 1253–1254); *If you strike it with a hammer a sound will be heard far away, like when one strikes a bronze frying pan* → "Ferez l'un poi, si orrez cler / Com si çoe fust metal soner" (Strike it a little bit, and you will hear it clearly sound as if it was metal.) (CL 1255–1256); *The one who wears it without being defiled through cohabitation will always have a pleasant voice* → "Qui chastement la portera, / A toz tens bone voiz avra." (He who wears it in chastity will always have a pleasant voice) (CL 1257–1258).

61. *robin*

Berakhyah gives no description of the *robin*, but refers to the **carbocle* (entry no. 53).

62. *saphir*

Berakhyah seems to have used multiple (partially unknown) sources. Maybe hence it follows that he brings the sapphire and the jacinth together—one being a variety of the other in Berakhyah's text—, so that first the amount of information becomes more abundant and ambiguous. Secondly, the *saphir*, considered as the generic term, gets three subcategories, i.e., it is firstly divided into the **saphir jacint*, the **wazzer saphir* and the **saphir orient*, from which the first one, the **jacint saphir*, is again divided into *jacint*, **wazzer jacint* and the unknown **alestre*. And here once more, for the third time, the first variety, the *jacint*, is split up into a granular, a spotted and a smooth kind. Schematically, the three levels of variation can be illustrated by the following table, which should be read top down:

Level			*saphir*		
1.		**saphir jacint*		**wazzer saphir*	**saphir orient*
2.	*jacint*	**wazzer jacint*	**alestre (?)*		
3.	*1. granular, 2. spotted, 3. smooth*				

The fact that he erroneously took the *jacint* for a variety of the **saphir jacint* instead of recognizing it as two names for one and the same stone, leads him to the assumption of third level of variation (the granular, the spotted and the smooth kinds of jacinth, cf. below).

Two stones—the **jagonce marine* and the **jacint grenat*—are mentioned separately from this scheme; they form indeed, together with the *(hyacinthus) citrinus*, the traditional division of the *hyacinthus* (cf. Marb. Red. lap. XIV, 214–215). Berakhyah seems to have had a Marbode source, but did not know where to place these two varieties of jacinth.

It remains unclear if with the **wazzer saphir*, the **wazzer jacint* and the **jagonce marine* the same stone, i.e., the water jacinth (*hyacinthus aquaticus*), is meant. The schematic table suggests three different stones, but in our sources, we could only find one kind: a variety of the jacinth.

a. saphir

We could find textual parallels in the Third Prose Lapidary and the Cambridge Lapidary. The comparison of the colour of the **saphir jacint* to the sky and the designation "oriental" of the **saphir orient* is present in the TP (cf. TP III), as well as the power of the *saphir* of keeping the limbs healthy and of setting free from chains (cf. loc. cit.). For the following issues, the CL was probably the source: *It alleviates external illnesses and it cools the fever of internal organs* → "Les mals del cors defors guarist; / Le chalt dedenz tost refreidist" (It cures external illness of the body; it cools internal fever in a short time.) (CL 177–178); *It appeases headache and stops sweating; it is beneficial for the eyes* → "Del chief a l'hume tolt dolur / E destreint forment la suur. / […] / As oelz ad ele grant mestier" (It appeases headache of men and stops [their] sweating well. It is very beneficial for the eyes.) (CL 181–184).

b. jacint

A combination of different Lat. and Angl.-Nor. texts may have been the source of Berakhyah for describing the *hyacinthus*. A similar differentiation between the three species of the *hyacinthus* can be found in Albertus Magnus: *[…] three species of the jacinth […]* → "[…] there are three names [i.e., *hyacinthus, aquaticus, saphirinus*]". (Albert. M. miner. II, 2, 8); *One is called jacinte; it is somewhat resembles the topaz* → "And some people say that there is a fourth kind green like *topasion*" (Albert. M. miner. II, 2, 17); *The second [species] is white as the seawater and it is called water jacinth* → "The 'water jacinth' is pale blue, as if the clearness of water welled up […]" (loc. cit.).

The virtue of the *jacint* of protecting against despondency and accidents as well as to change its colour according to the weather can also be found in the CL (cf. CL 363–376), whereas the three kinds: granular, spotted and smooth only figure in the Alphabetic Lapidary: *Moreover, the jacinth which is called jacinte is divided into three [kinds]. One is granular, the second is all covered with bright spots, and the third is smooth* → "Jacintus est de pere nom, / De treis maneres la trovum: / Grain ad en l'une, en l'autre vaines, / E la tierce manere est plaine" (*Jacintus* is the name of this stone, which we find in three kinds: one of them is granular, another has veins, and the third kind is smooth.) (AL 1231–1234). Finally, the faculty of the **jagonce marine* of cooling a feverish body can be found in the First Prose Lapidary (cf. FP X).

63. *solenite*

The Cambridge Version of Marbode seems to be the source for the *solenite*: *Its hue is like honey, somewhat tending towards green* → "Com herbe verz est sa color" (Its colour is like green herb.) (CL 669); *When the Moon waxes, it increases and when it wanes, it decreases* → "Croist et descroist solonc la lune" (It increases and decreases in accordance with the Moon.) (CL 673); *He who wears it will attract the love of the people* → "Mult bone est sor soi a porter / Por amor d'omes recovrer" (It is very good to wear it for regaining the love of the people.) (CL 677–678); *It possesses this virtue [only] when the moon waxes* → "Mais ke si soit ke al croissant / La portent a lor col pendant" (But if you want this to happen, you have to wear it around your neck when the Moon waxes.) (CL 683–684).

64. *sardine*

A definite source for the *sardine* could not be identified. However, the following parallels, taken from the Angl.-Nor. Marbode versions (First Prose Lapidary and Verse Adaption), are noteworthy: *Its [hue] is ⟨between⟩ reddish and red. It is very beautiful. However, it is has not the power of [...]* → "Ele est ruge [...]. Ele n'ad nule vertud fors la bealtéd" (It is red. It has no virtues except for its beauty.) (FP XLVII); *[...] it appeases bad dreams* → "Tuz vains pensers de li s'en fuit" (All dark thoughts disappear from him [i.e. from the one who wears it].) (VA 484).

65. *sardonice*

For this stone, two Angl.-Nor. Marbode versions could be a possible source of Berakhyah's description, i.e., the Cambridge Version and the First Prose Lapidary. Its composition of two names is explained in the CL: *It has two names [...]* → "Il est de dous nuns cumposez, / Çoe est d'oniche et de sardine" (It is composed of two names, namely the *oniche* and the *sardine*.) (CL 248–249); the reference to the higher esteem of the dark kind of the stone is also present there: *The dark [dull] [stone] is better than the pure [brilliant] one* → "Cum plus est oscur et mielz valt" (The darker it is, the higher it is esteemed.) (CL 261). The detailled description of its physical aspect corresponds better to the description given in the FP: *[…] white upon black, and black upon white. […]. Its hue is purple […]. When [the stone] has both colours [clearly distinguished] next to the black, then [the stone] is good: you then see the white, and above it red which is like blood* → "[…] le blaunc i est sur le neir et le ruge sur le blaunc. […] cele ki les treis culurs ad bien devisees e nient entremellees, cele est la mielz preisede." (White is there upon black, and red upon white. The one which has the three colours well distinguished and not intermixed, this one is the most esteemed.) (FP VI).

66. *serpentine*

No sources could be identified for the *serpentine* (cf. section 2).

67. *sadde*

For this stone, we can again identify the Cambridge Lapidary as Berakhyah's source. The comparison of its colour with the one of the *prame* (i.e., the green prase) features—beneath in the CL (cf. CL 918–919)—in the First French Version (cf. FF 690) as well, but the remark that the *sadde* is a precious stone can only be found in the CL (cf. CL 899). Moreover, the spelling of the Hebrew term corresponds with the one in the CL (*sadde* in CL 899 in contrast to *sade* in FF 683). For Berakhyah's information that the stone is a kind of turquoise, no source could be retrieved.

For stones nos. 68–70, which have Hebrew names, an unknown Hebrew source is assumed by the authors (cf. the introduction).

71. *cilidonia*

The First French Version of Marbode is, in all probability, the source for Berakhyah's description of this stone, since we find very close textual parallels and the reference to most of its virtues:

*It can be found in a bird called *aradnela (arondele) [namely] in its intestines […]* → "El ventre creist de l'arundele" (It is generated in the stomach of the swallow.) (FF 396); *Two kinds [of this stone] exist: one is entirely black or has black spots; and there is a red one* → "Dient k'el est de dous maneres, / Dous sunt trové, de dous culurs: / L'un trait al neir, l'altr' a rovurs" (They say that it is found in two varieties; two [kinds] are found, with two different colours: One tends towards black, the other towards red.) (FF 398–400); *The red one is very beneficial for those who have an epileptic [fit] with the New Moon* → "La ruige toilt la passiun / Ke prent a ume par luneisun, / [...]" (The red one cures epilepsy, which affects men with the moon.) (FF 401–402); *The one who wears it, should wrap it in a white, clean linen garment and put that garment in a honey-coloured pouch, and hang it on his left side* → "En linge drap seit volopee / E al senestre bras portee" (It should be wrapped in a linen sheet and worn on the left arm.) (FF 407–408); *Then he will find favour in the eyes of all those who see him* → "Celui ki l'a fait bien parler / E mult de tute gent amer" (It makes the one who has it speak well and beloved by everyone.) (FF 405–406); *With the black [variety] one should proceed in the same way* → "En meisme ceste manere / S'est portee la neire piere" (In the same way one should proceed [regarding] the black stone.) (FF 409–410); *He who carries it on him [...] will not be affected by strife, for it soothes even the wrath of the king* → "E defent ume de cuntraire; / Cuntre ire de prinze e de reis / dune force, aïe e defeis" (And it protects you against hostility; it gives you strength, it helps [you] and protects [you] against the wrath of princes and kings.) (FF 412–414); *He who washes his eyes with water in which the stone had been immersed, his eyes will be cured from many diseases* → "L'eue u ceste piere est lavee / Saine les oilz de la bobee" (The water in which the stone has been washed heals the eyes from eye diseases.) (FF 415–416); *Someone who suffers from a fever or from [superfluous] humour should carry it on him* → "Iceste piere [...] / Toilt fevre e les males umurs [...]" (This stone removes fever and harmful humours.) (FF 418–419).

72. *ceraune*

The information about the *ceraune* is mostly taken from the Cambridge Version of Marbode. However, the statement of Berakhyah that the stone is also called "thunderstone" does not go back to the Pliny—Isidore—Marbode tradition, where the name of the stone is always explained by its origin in lightning strikes. Actually, the Gr. etymon of the *ceraune*, κεραυνός, means both, lightning and thunder (cf. LS 942a). As far as we could see, Albertus Magnus is the only author who relates the stone to thunder: "It is said to fall sometimes from a cloud with the thunder" (Albert. M. miner. II, 2, 3). Analogically, he mentions below the virtue of the stone "[of protecting] against the danger of thunder" (loc. cit.), whereas Berakhyah notes the protective power against the harm of both lightning and thunder; cf. for the protection againts lightning, e.g., the CL: "La fuldre ne li fera mal, / Ki la porte chastement; / En toz leus tot ensement / [...] / Ja nule fuldre n'i charra" (He who wears it in chastity will not be harmed by lightnings; wherever [it is], no lightning will thus strike.) (CL 714–719).

For the other issues, the CL comes very close: *Its colour is somewhat similar to crystal* → "Par pou ne semble cristal" (It is somewhat similar to crystal.) (CL 713); *If it is carried in a ship, the latter will not sink or wrack, and the wind will not harm it* → "Ne la nef ki curra par mer / Ne puet brisier ne reverser, / Ne mal ne li fera nus venz, / ou ceste piere iert dedenz" (Neither the ship that is at sea can sink or wreck, nor the wind can harm it, if this stone is aboard the ship.) (CL 721–724); *It is beneficial for [...] becoming victorious in war* → "E en bataille ki l'avra, / Trestoz ses enemis vaintra." (He who wears it in battle, will defeat all his enemies.) (CL 725–726); *He who wears it while lying down, will have good dreams* → "Ki dolz sunges velt sungier, / Od soi la porte a son cuchier." (He who wants to have sweet dreams, should wear it when he goes to bed.) (CL 727–728); *There are two varieties: one is similar to flame and the other looks like ice* → "De cestes precioses pieres / poet l'en trover de dous manires; / [...] / L'une est blanche cume glace, / L'autre est un petit galnace." (You can find two varieties of [this precious stone]: one is white like ice, the other is somewhat yellowish.) (CL 729–736).

4. *Tables of the Sources*

The following tables show on the left side the sources that we could identify (abbreviations explained in the footnotes) with the pertinent stones on the corresponding right side. Angl.-Nor. and Lat. sources are presented in separate tables; descriptions of stones with uncertain sources are labeled with a question mark.

This overview makes it possible to determine very quickly the primary source of Berakhyah: the Angl.-Nor. Cambridge Version of Marbode, which was probably used as source for 44 (out of 72) stones. Secondary and uncertain[85] sources follow further below in the tables, arranged in the order of their supposed importance for Berakhyah.

[85] Especially texts with three and less pertinent stones can be called in question as source.

4.1. *Anglo-Norman Source Texts*

Source text	Pertinent stones
CL[86]	*aimant (1), alectoire (3), esmeralde (4), onicle (5), etite (6), heliotrope (7), ematis (9), abeste (10), exacontalithos (11), orite (12), enidre (13), alemandine (15), yenia (16), iris (17), androdragma (18), optallie (19), absite (20), beril (28), grisolite (29), grisopacion (31), gagatromé (32), galactites (33), gelazias (35), diadocode (36), dionise (37), diamant (38), jaiet (42), gerachite (43), gelazia (44)?, ligurie (46), medus (47), pantera (49), pedoretes (50), carboncle (53), coral (54), cornoligne (56), cristal (57), calcofone (60), saphir (62), jacint (62), solenite (63), sardonice (65), sadde (67), ceraune (72)*
FF[87]	*acates (2), onicle (5), ametiste (14), grisolite (29), diamant (38), jaiet (42), perle (48)?, carboncle (53), calcidonia (58), cilidonia (71)*
AL[88]	*acates (2), onicle (5), alemandine (15), beril (28), grisolite (29), gelazias (35), colire (55), jacint (62)*
FP[89]	*aimant (1), grisolite (29), ligurie (46), jacinte (62), sardine (64)?, sardonice (65)*
SP[90]	*aimant (1), ametiste (14), jaspe (41), pantera (49)*
TP[91]	*esmeralde (4), diamant (38), jaiet (42), saphir (62)*
VA[92]	*topace (40)?, ligurie (46), carboncle (53)*
AP[93]	*grisopras (30)*
Meyer 1909	*ancotre (23)?*

[86] CL = Cambridge Version (ed. Studer & Evans 1924).
[87] FF = First French Version (ed. Studer & Evans 1924).
[88] AL = Alphabetical Lapidary (ed. Studer & Evans 1924).
[89] FP = First Prose Lapidary (ed. Studer & Evans 1924).
[90] FP = First Prose Lapidary (ed. Studer & Evans 1924).
[91] TP = Third Prose Lapidary (ed. Studer & Evans 1924).
[92] VA = Verse Adaption (ed. Studer & Evans 1924).
[93] AP = Apocalyptical Lapidary (ed. Studer & Evans 1924).

4.2. *Latin Source Texts*

Source text	Pertinent stones
Isidore[94]	*electrum (21), optallius (22), ancotre (23)?, asterites (26), legnete (45)*
Albertus Magnus[95]	*electrum (21), coral (54), camahieu (59)?, jacint (62)*
Damigeron[96]	*optallius (22), legnete (45), coral (54)*
Pliny[97]	*electrum (21), legnete (45)*
Digby 13[98]	*coral (54)*
Marbode[99]	*calcidonia (58)*

[94] Isid. nat. orig. XVI (ed. Lindsay 1911).
[95] Albert. M. miner. (transl. Wyckoff 1976).
[96] Damig. lap. (ed. Abel 1881).
[97] Plin. nat. XXXVII (ed. König 1979).
[98] MS. Bodleian Digby 13 (in MJE, ed. Evans 1922).
[99] Marb. Red. lap. (ed. Riddle 1977).

ALPHABETICAL GLOSSARIES

1. *Hebrew—French/Latin/Greek Glossary*

Stone no.	French/Latin/Greek	Hebrew
1	*aimant*	אַאִימַנְט
7	*heliotrope*	אאליוטרופא
8	*abeste*	אַבִישְׁטא
10	*abeste*	אַבֵישְׁט
20	*absite*	אַבשִׁיטַא
30	**ortice (artetice)*	אוירטץ
5	*onicle*	אוניקלא
22	**uptalus (optallius)*	אֻופטלוּש
19	**optallies (optallie)*	אוֹפטליאש
6	*occian*	אוֹקצִיַאן
12	*orite*	אוֹרֵיטא
9	**ematice (ematite)*	אֵימַטִיש
6	*etite*	אִיטִיטְא
14	**ematice (ametiste)*	אֵימַטִישְׁא
16	*hyaena*	איניאה
16	*yenia*	אֵינִיאַה
11	**exacratlitu (exacontalithus)*	אֵיקְשַקְרַטְלִיטו
17	**irone (iris)*	אירונא
17	**irone (iris)*	אִירוֹנְא
26	*asterites*	אֵישְׁטְרִיטַש
3	**alectuine (alectoire)*	אַלֵיקְטוּיינְא
21	*electrum*	אֵלִיקְטְרום
15	*alemandine*	אַלְמְדִינְא
14	ἆιμα	אֵמַה
27	**amauntes (amiantus)*	אַמַאֻונְטְש
18	**andro dragaza (androdragma)*	אַנדְרוֹ דְרַגַצַא
13	*enidre*	אַנִידְרְא
23	**ancotre*	אַנְקוטְרא
25	**ansra (ambra)*	אַנְסְרַא
24	**asistos*	אַסִצְטוּש
38	*ascier*	אַצִיר
2	*acates*	אקטץ
71	**aradnela (arondele)*	אַרַדנלא

4, 39	*esmeralde*	אֵשמרַלדְא
25	*baleine*	בַלֵינְא
28	*beril*	בֵירֵיל
32	*gagatromé*	גַגַטרֹום
52	*gote crampe*	גוטא קרנפא
39	*jaiet*	גֵייטְא
34	**galictotea*	גַלִיקְטוֹטְיַא
33	*galactites*	גַלַקְטִיטַש
35	*gelazias*	גְלַקְצִיאַש
44	*gresil*	גרזיל
29	*grisolite*	גְרִיזוּלֵיט
30	*grisoprase*	גְרִיזוֹפְרֶש
31	**grisopacion (crisopacion)*	גרישופציאון
37	*dionise*	דְאוֹנִיש
1, 38	*diamant*	דִיאַמַנְט
36	*diadocode*	דִיאַדְקוּדְא
46	*date*	דֵיטְא
39	*venes*	וינש
62	**wazzer saphir (jagunce evage)*	וַשְר שפיר
62	**wazzer jacant (jagunce evage)*	ושר יכנט
62	*topace*	טופסא
40	*topace*	טוֹפַסְא
39	**torquois (turquois)*	טוֹרְקְוִיש
42	*jaiet*	יאייט
62	**jagunce marine (jagunce evage)*	יגונצא מרינא
44	**gelaza (gelazia)*	יִילַצַא
62	*jacint*	יכנט
62	**jacant (jacint)*	יַכַנְט
62	**jacint grenat (jagonce grenat)*	יכנט גרנט
62	**jacite (jacinte)*	יסיטא
43	*gerachite*	יַרַיִיטא
41	*jaspe*	יַשְפְא
46	*ligurie*	לִיגוֹרֵיאַה
45	**legnete*	לִינֵיטְא
1	*magnetes*	מַגְנֵיטִיש
47	**medo (medus)*	מֵידו
62	*milfoil*	מילפוייל
48	*margarite*	מרגריטא
62	**alestre*	עלישטרא
4	**porels (porreus)*	פורלש
3	*feve*	פיבא
50	*pedoretes*	פִידוֹרַטַש
51	**paitoros*	פַיְיטוֹרוֹש
48	*perle*	פֵירְלְא
49	*pantera*	פַנְטֵירַא
52	**peritora*	פְרִיטוֹרַא
67	**prime (prame)*	פרימא

14	*pesques*	פֵּישְׁקְש
14	**zonce (jagonce) grenat*	צונצא גרנט
71	*cilidonia*	צִילִידוֹנְיַא
71	*cipres*	צִיפַּרְש
68	*ceraune*	צירוניא
72	**ceriaun (ceraune)*	צֵירִיאוֹן
55	*colire*	קוֹלֵירַא
9	**collyriu (collyrium)*	קולירי͏ו
56	**cortolina (cornoligne)*	קוֹרְטוֹלִינַא
2	*coral*	קוֹרָל
54	*coral*	קוֹרַל
58	*calcidonia*	קַלְצִידוֹנְיַא
60	**calcofine (calcofone)*	קַלקופִינְא
59	**camahu (camahieu)*	קַמַהוּ
53	*carboncle*	קַרְבּוֹקְלא
2	*Crete*	קַרֵיטְא
62	*cristal*	קרישטל
57	*cristal*	קְרִישְׁטַל
64	*crampe*	קרנפא
53	*robin*	רובין
61	*robin*	רוֹבִּין
4	**Ciie (Cithie)*	שאיאה
63	*solenite*	שׁוֹלְנִיטֵי
2	*Sezile*	שְׁזִילְא
62	*saphir*	שפיר
62	**saphir orient*	שפיר אוריאנט
62	**saphir jacint (jargunce saphire)*	שפיר יַכַנְט
67	*sadde*	שדד
14	*sarde*	שֵׂרְדְא
65	**sarde onique (sardonice)*	שַׂרְדַא אוֹנִיקַא
5, 64	*sardine*	שַׂרְדִינְא
66	*serpentine*	שרפנטינא

2. *French/Latin—Hebrew Glossary*

French/Latin	Hebrew	Stone no.
abeste	אַבִישְׁטא, אַבֵישְׁט	8, 10
absite	אַבשִׁיטַא	20
acates	אקטץ	2
aimant	אַאִימַנְט	1
*alectoire (*alectuine)*	אַלֵיקְטוּיְינְא	3
alemandine	אַלְמְדִינְא	15
**alestre*	עלישטרא	62
*ambra (*ansra)*	אַנְסְרַא	25

*ametiste (*ametice)*	אֵימַטִישְׁא	14
*amianthus (*amauntes)*	אַמַאֻונְטְש	27
**ancotre*	אַנְקוֹטְרא	23
*androdragma (*andro dragaza)*	אַנדְּרוֹ דְרַגַצַא	18
*arondele (*aradnela)*	אַרַדנלא	71
*artetice (*ortice)*	אוירטץ	30
ascier	אַצִיר	38
**asistos*	אַסִצְטוּש	24
asterites	אֵישְׁטְרִיטַש	26
baleine	בַלֵינְא	25
beril	בֵירֵיל	28
calcidonia	קַלְצִידוֹנְיַא	58
*calcofone (*calcofine)*	קַלקופִינְא	60
*camahieu (*camahu)*	קַמַהוּ	59
carboncle	קַרְבוֹקְלא	53
ceraune	צירוניא	68
*ceraune (*ceriaun)*	צֵירִיאוֹן	72
cilidonia	צִילִידוֹנְיַא	71
cipres	צִיפַרש	71
*Cithie (*Ciie)*	שאיאה	4
colire	קוֹלֵירַא	55
*collyrium (*collyriu)*	קוליריו	9
coral	קוֹרַל ,קוּרָל	2, 54
*cornoligne (*cortolina)*	קוֹרְטוֹלִינַא	56
crampe	קרנפא	64
Crete	קַרֵיטְא	2
*crisopacion (*grisopacion)*	גרישופציאון	31
cristal	קרישטל, קְרִישְׁטַל	57, 62
date	דֵיטְא	46
diadocode	דיאַדְקודְא	36
diamant	דִיאַמַנְט	38
dionise	דְאוֹנִיש	37
electrum	אֵלִיקְטְרום	21
*ematite (*ematice)*	אֵימַטִיש	9
enidre	אַנִידְרְא	13
esmeralde	אֵשמַרַלדְא	4, 39
etite	אִיטִיטְא	6
*exacontalithus (*exacratlitu)*	אֵיקְשַקְרַטְלִיטו	11
feve	פיבא	3
gagatromé	גַגַטרוֹם	32
galactites	גַלַקְטִיטַש	33
**galictotea*	גַלִיקְטוֹטְיַא	34
gelazias	גְלַקְצִיאַש	35
*gelazia (*gelaza)*	יִילַצַא	44
gerachite	יַרַיִיטא	43
gote crampe	גוטא קרנפא	52
gresil	גרזיל	44

grisolite	גְרִיזוֹלֵיט	29
grisoprase	גְרִיזוֹפְרְש	30
heliotrope	אאליוטרופא	7
hyaena	איניאה	16
*iris (*irone)*	אִירוֹנְא	17
**irone*	אירונא	17
jacint	יכנט	62
*jacint (*jacant)*	יַכַנְט,	62
*jacinte (*jacite)*	יסיטא	62
*jagunce evage (*wazzer saphir)*	וַושְר שפיר	62
*(*wazzer jacant)*	ושר יכנט	62
*(*jagunce marine)*	יגונצא מרינא	62
*jagonce grenat (*jacint grenat)*	יכנט גרנט	62
*jagonce grenat (*zonce grenat)*	צונצא גרנט	14
jaiet	גֵייטְא, יאייט	39, 42
*jargunce saphire (*saphir jacint)*	שפיר יַכַנְט	62
jaspe	יַשְפְא	41
**legnete*	לְינֵיטְא	45
ligurie	לִיגוֹרֵיאַה	46
magnetes	מַגְנֵיטְיש	1
margarite	מרגריטא	48
*medus (*medo)*	מֵידו	47
milfoil	מילפוייל	62
occian	אוֹקצִיַאן	6
onicle	אניקלא	5
*optallie (*optallies)*	אופטליאש	19
*optallius (*uptalus)*	אֻופטלוּש	22
orite	אוֹרֵיטא	12
**paitoros*	פַייטוֹרוֹש	51
pantera	פַנְטֵירַא	49
pedoretes	פִידוֹרַטַש	50
**peritora*	פְרִיטוֹרַא	52
perle	פֵירְלְא	48
pesques	פֵרשְקְש	14
*porreus (*porels)*	פורלש	4
*prame (*prime)*	פרימא	67
robin	רוֹבִין, רובין	53, 61
saphir	שפיר	62
**saphir orient*	שפיר אוריאנט	62
sadde	שדד	67
sarde	שֵרְדְא	14
sardine	שַרְדִינְא	5, 64
*sardonice (*sarde onique)*	שַרְדַא אוֹנִיקַא	65
serpentine	שרפנטינא	66
Sezile	שְזִילְא	2
solenite	שוֹלְנִיטֵי	63
topace	טוֹפַסְא, טופסא	40, 62

*turquois (*torquois)*	טֹורְקֻוִיש	39
venes	וינש	39
yenia	אֵינְיאַה	16

3. *Greek—Hebrew Glossary*

Greek	Hebrew	Stone no.
ἆιμα	אֵמַה	14

BIBLIOGRAPHY AND ABBREVIATIONS

AL = "The Alphabetical Lapidary", in: *Anglo-Norman Lapidaries*, ed. Studer, Paul & Joan Evans (1924). Paris: Champion, pp. 200–259 [reprint Genève 1976].

Albertus Magnus, *Book of Minerals*, transl. by Wyckoff, Dorothy (1976). Oxford: Clarendon Press.

AND = *Anglo-Norman Dictionary*, ed. Stone, Louise W. & William Rothwell (1977–1992), 7 vols. London: The Modern Humanities Research Association.

AP = "The Apocalyptic Lapidary", in: *Anglo-Norman Lapidaries*, ed. Studer, Paul & Joan Evans (1924). Paris: Champion, pp. 260–276 [reprint Genève 1976].

Aslanov, Cyril (2001): *Le provençal des juifs et l'hébreu en Provence: le dictionnaire Sarsot ha-Kesef de Joseph Caspi*. Paris: Peeters.

Banitt, Menahem (1963): "Une langue fantôme: le judéo-français", in: *Revue de Linguistique Romane* 27, pp. 245–294.

Banitt, Menahem (1971): "Judéo-French", in: *Encyclopaedia Judaica*, vol. 10, pp. 423–425. Jerusalem: Macmillan.

Blondheim, David Simon (1925): *Les parlers judéo-romans et la Vetus Latina. Etude sur les rapports entre les traductions bibliques en langue romane des Juifs au Moyen Age et les anciennes versions*. Paris: Champion.

Blondheim, David Simon (1927): *Poèmes judéo-français du Moyen Age*. Paris: Champion.

Bos, Gerrit & Guido Mensching (2001): "Shem Ṭov Ben Isaac, Glossary of Botanical Terms, Nos. 1–18", in: *The Jewish Quarterly Review XCII/1–2*, pp. 21–40.

Bos, Gerrit & Guido Mensching (2005): "The Literature of Hebrew Medical Synonyms: Romance and Latin Terms and Their Identification". In: *Aleph* 5, pp. 169–211.

Bos, Gerrit & Guido Mensching (forthcoming): *A Glossary of Medico-Botanical Terms. The 29th Book of Sefer ha-Šimmuš by Shem Ṭov Ben Isaac of Tortosa.*

CL = "The Cambridge Version of Marbode's Lapidary", in: *Anglo-Norman Lapidaries*, ed. Studer, Paul & Joan Evans (1924). Paris: Champion, pp. 154–199 [reprint Genève 1976].

Dalven, Rachel (1971): "Judeo-Greek", in: *Encyclopaedia Judaica*, vol. 10, pp. 425–427. Jerusalem: Macmillan.

Damigeron, *De lapidibus*, ed. Abel, Eugenius (1881). Berlin: Calvary, digital version of the reprint [Hildesheim 1971] by Gloning, Thomas (URL on 9/27 2007: http://www.uni-giessen.de/gloning/tx/damig3.htm).

DAO = *Dictionnaire onomasiologique de l'ancien occitan*, ed. by Baldinger, Kurt (1975–), 9- fasc. Tübingen: Niemeyer.

DB = Darmesteter, Arsène & David S. Blondheim (1929): *Les Gloses françaises dans les commentaires talmudiques de Raschi*, 1st vol. Paris: Champion.

DCVB = Alcover, A.M. / Moll, F. de B. (1935): *Diccionari català-valencià-balear*, vol. 1: *A-ARQ* (1930), vol. 2: *ARR-CAR*. Palma de Mallorca: Moll.

DETEMA = *Diccionario español de textos médicos antiguos*, ed. by Maria Teresa Herrera (1996), 2 vols. Madrid: Arco Libros.

DHLP = *Dicionário Honaiss da língua portuguesa*, ed. by Antônio Honaiss et al. (2001). Rio de Janeiro: Objetiva.

FEW = *Französisches Etymologisches Wörterbuch. Eine Darstellung des galloromanischen Sprachschatzes*, ed. by Walter von Wartburg (1922–), 25- vols. Bonn/ Heidelberg/ Leipzig/ Basel.

Fischel, Walter Joseph (1971): "Judeo-Persian", in: *Encyclopaedia Judaica*, vol. 10, pp. 429–432. Jerusalem: Macmillan.

FF = "The First French Version of Marbode's Lapidary", in: *Anglo-Norman Lapidaries*, ed. Studer, Paul & Joan Evans (1924). Paris: Champion, pp. 19–69 [reprint Genève 1976].

FP = "First Anglo-Norman Prose Lapidary", in: *Anglo-Norman Lapidaries*, ed. Studer, Paul & Joan Evans (1924). Paris: Champion, pp. 97–111 [reprint Genève 1976].

GDLI = *Grande dizionario della lingua italiana*, ed. by Salvatore Battaglia (1961–2009), 24 vols. Turin: Unione.

GH = Georges, Karl Ernst ([8]1913–1918): *Ausführliches Lateinisch-Deutsches Handwörterbuch*, 2 vols. Hannover/ Leipzig: Hahnsche Buchhandlung.

Goltz, Dietlinde (1972): *Studien zur Geschichte der Mineralnamen in Pharmazie, Chemie und Medizin von den Anfängen bis Paracelsus*. Wiesbaden: Steiner.

Halkin, Abraham Solomon (1971): "Judeo-Arabic Literature", in: *Encyclopaedia Judaica*, vol. 10, pp. 410–423. Jerusalem: Macmillan.

Isidorus Hispalensis, *Etymologiarum sive originum libri XX*, ed. Lindsay, W.M. (1911), vol. 2 (libros XI–XX continens). Oxford: University Press.

Katzenellenbogen, Lucie (1933): *Eine altfranzösische Abhandlung über Fieber* (doctoral thesis). Würzburg: Triltsch.

Kiwitt, Marc (2001): *Der altfranzösische Fiebertraktat Fevres. Teiledition und sprachwissenschaftliche Untersuchung*. Würzburg: Königshausen & Neumann.

Kramer, Johannes & Sabine Kowallik (1994): *Einführung in die hebräische Schrift*. Hamburg: Buske.

Kramer, Johannes (1996): "Verschriftungsarten und -tendenzen in der Romania", in: *Lexikon der romanistischen Linguistik*, vol. 2,1, pp. 584–597. Tübingen: Niemeyer.

Levy, Raphael (1932): *Recherches lexicographiques sur d'ancien textes français d'origine juive*. Baltimore: John Hopkins Press.

Levy, Raphael (1964): *Trésor de la langue des Juifs au Moyen Age*. Austin/ London: University of Texas Press.

LTL = *Lexicon Toutius Latinitatis*, ed. by Egidio Forcellini ([2]1965). Bononiae: Forni.

LS = Liddell, Henry George ([9]1996): *A Greek-English Lexicon*. With a revised supplement by Henry George Liddell and Robert Scott, revised and augmented throughout by Henry Stuart Jones. Oxford: Clarendon.

Lexer, Matthias ([38]1992): *Mittelhochdeutsches Taschenwörterbuch*. Stuttgart: Hirzel.

Marbodus of Rennes, *De lapidibus, Considered as a Medical Treatise with Text, Commentary and C.W. King's Translation, together with text and translation of Marbode's Minor Works on Stones*, ed. Riddle, John M. (1977). Wiesbaden: Steiner.

Menger, Louis Emil (1904): *The Anglo-Norman Dialect. A Manual of its Phonology and Morphology with Illustrative Specimens of the Literature*. New York: Columbia University Press / London: Macmillan.

Mensching, Guido & Frank Savelsberg (2004): "Reconstrucció de la terminologia mèdica occitanocatalana dels segles XIII i XIV a través de llistats de sinònims en lletres hebrees", in: *Actes del congrés per a l'estudi dels Jueus en territori de llengua catalana*, Barcelona-Girona 2001, pp. 69–81. Universidad de Barcelona.

Meyer, Paul (1909): "Les plus anciens lapidaires français (3e article)", in: *Romania XXXVIII*, pp. 481–552.

MJE = Evans, Joan (1922): *Magical Jewels of the Middle Ages and the Renaissance particularly in England*. Oxford: Clarendon [reprint New York 1976].

MLWB = *Mittellateinisches Wörterbuch bis zum ausgehenden 13. Jahrhundert*, ed. by Paul Lehmann, 3- vols. München: Beck.

Müller, Bodo (1975): *Das Französische der Gegenwart. Varietäten, Strukturen, Tendenzen*. Heidelberg: Winter.

ODEE = Onions, Charles T. (ed.) (1978): *The Oxford Dictionary of English Etymology*. Repr. with correcctions. Oxford: Clarendon.

Oesterreicher, Josef (1896): *Beiträge zur Geschichte der jüdisch-französischen Sprache und Literatur im Mittelalter*. Czernowitz: Pardini.

PL = "The Peterborough Lapidary", in: *English Medieval Dictionaries*, ed. Evans. Joan & Mary S. Serjeantson (1933). London: Oxford Universitiy Press.

Plinius Secundus, Gaius: *Naturalis historiae libri XXXVII*, ed. and transl. (ger.) by König, Roderich, vol. XXXVII (1979). Darmstadt: WBG.

Pope, Mildred K. (1934): *From Latin to Modern French with especial consideration of Anglo-Norman*. Manchester: Manchester University Press [reprint London 1952].

REW = *Romanisches etymologisches Wörterbuch*, ed. by Wilhelm Meyer-Lübke ([6]1992). Heidelberg: Winter.

Rheinfelder, Hans (1963): *Altfranzösische Grammatik*. First part: Phonology. München: Hueber.

Rheinfelder, Hans (1967): *Altfranzösische Grammatik*. Second part: Morphology. München: Hueber.

Sala, Marius (1998): "Die romanischen Judensprachen", in: *Lexikon der Romanistischen Linguistik*, vol. 7, pp. 372–395. Tübingen: Niemeyer.

Sin. = Mensching, Guido (1994): *La sinonima delos nonbres delas medeçinas griegos e latynos e arauigos. Estudio y edición crítica*. Madrid: Arco Libros.

Studer, Paul & Joan Evans (1924): *Anglo-Norman Lapidaries*. Paris: Champion [reprint Genève 1976].

SP = "Second Anglo-Norman Prose Lapidary", in: *Anglo-Norman Lapidaries*, ed. Studer, Paul & Joan Evans (1924). Paris: Champion, pp. 111–136 [reprint Genève 1976].

ThLL = *Thesaurus Linguae Latinae*, 10- vols. 1900–1999: Stuttgart/ Leipzig: Teubner; 2000–2006: Munich/ Leipzig: Sauer; since 2007: Berlin/ New York: de Gruyter.

TL = Tobler, Adolf & Erhard Lommatzsch (1925–1976): *Altfranzösisches Wörterbuch*, 11 vols. Vols. 1–10: Berlin/ Wiesbaden, vol. 11 (ed. by Hans Helmut Christmann 1989): Stuttgart.

TP = "Third Anglo-Norman Prose Lapidary", in: *Anglo-Norman Lapidaries*, ed. Studer, Paul & Joan Evans (1924). Paris: Champion, pp. 136–153 [reprint Genève 1976].

VA = "Anglo-Norman Verse Adaption of the 'First French Version' and Fragments of Other Verse translations of Marbode's Poem", in: *Anglo-Norman Lapidaries*, ed. Studer, Paul & Joan Evans (1924). Paris: Champion, pp. 71–93 [reprint Genève 1976].

Vossler, Karl (1929): *Frankreichs Kultur und Sprache*. Heidelberg: Winter.

Weinreich, Max (1956): "The Jewish Languages of Romance Stock and their Relation to Earliest Yiddish", in: *Romance Philology* 9, pp. 403–428.

Wexler, Paul (1981): "The Jewish Interlinguistics: Facts and Conceptual Framework", in: *Language* 57, pp. 99–149.

Zaun, Stefanie (2002): "Fieberbehandlung im Mittelalter. Edition und Analyse eines altfranzösischen Textes in hebräischer Graphie", in: *Konzepte der Nation: Eingrenzung, Ausgrenzung, Entgrenzung*, ed. by Schleicher, Regina & Almut Wilske, pp. 273–291. Bonn: Romanistischer Verlag.

Zwink, Julia (unedited): *Ein altfranzösischer Fiebertraktat in hebräischer Graphie (Staatsbibliothek zu Berlin—Preußischer Kulturbesitz, Ms. or. oct. 512): Edition und Analyse ausgewählter Passagen* (Master's thesis).

Zwink, Julia (2006): "Étude lexicographique du traité anonyme Fevres: Une compilation médicale en ancien français, écrite en caractères hébraïques", in: *Panace@* 24, pp. 250–260 (online: http://www.medtrad.org/panacea/IndiceGeneral/n24_tribunahistorica-zwink.pdf).

SUBJECT INDEX OF ENGLISH AND FOREIGN TERMS

The numbers refer to the sections of the English translation.

PLATES

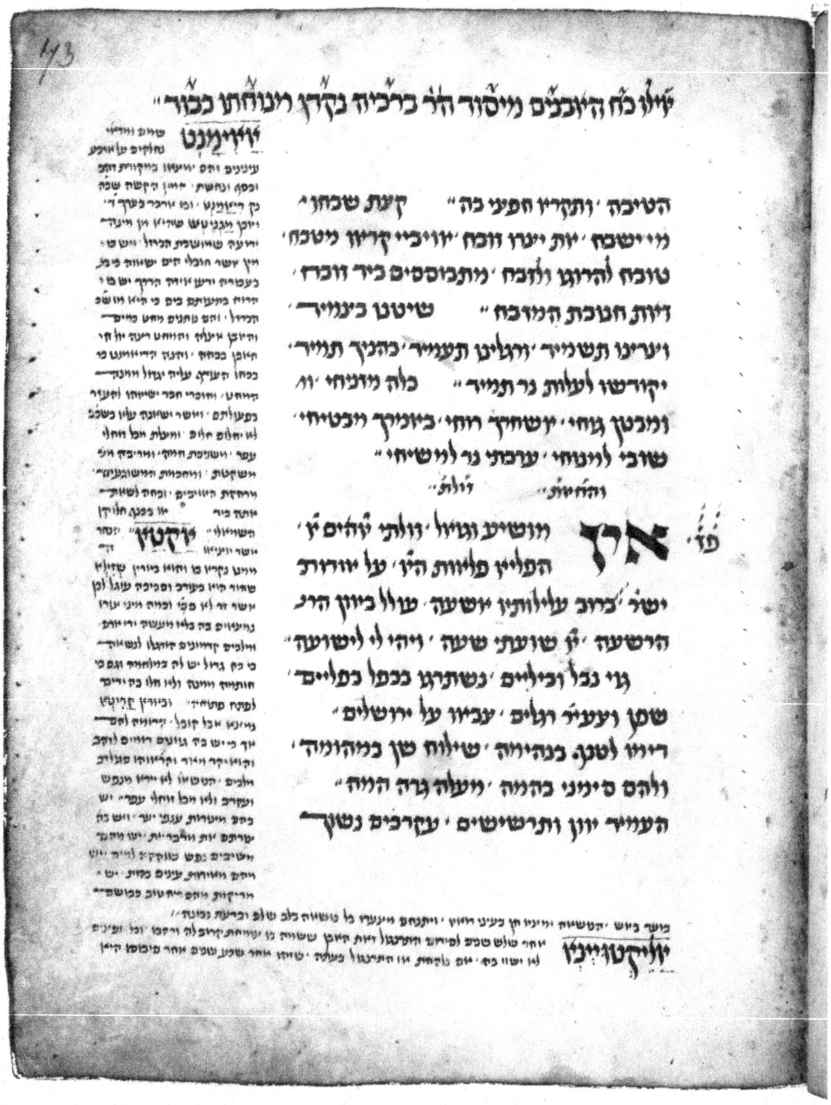

1. fol. 73r

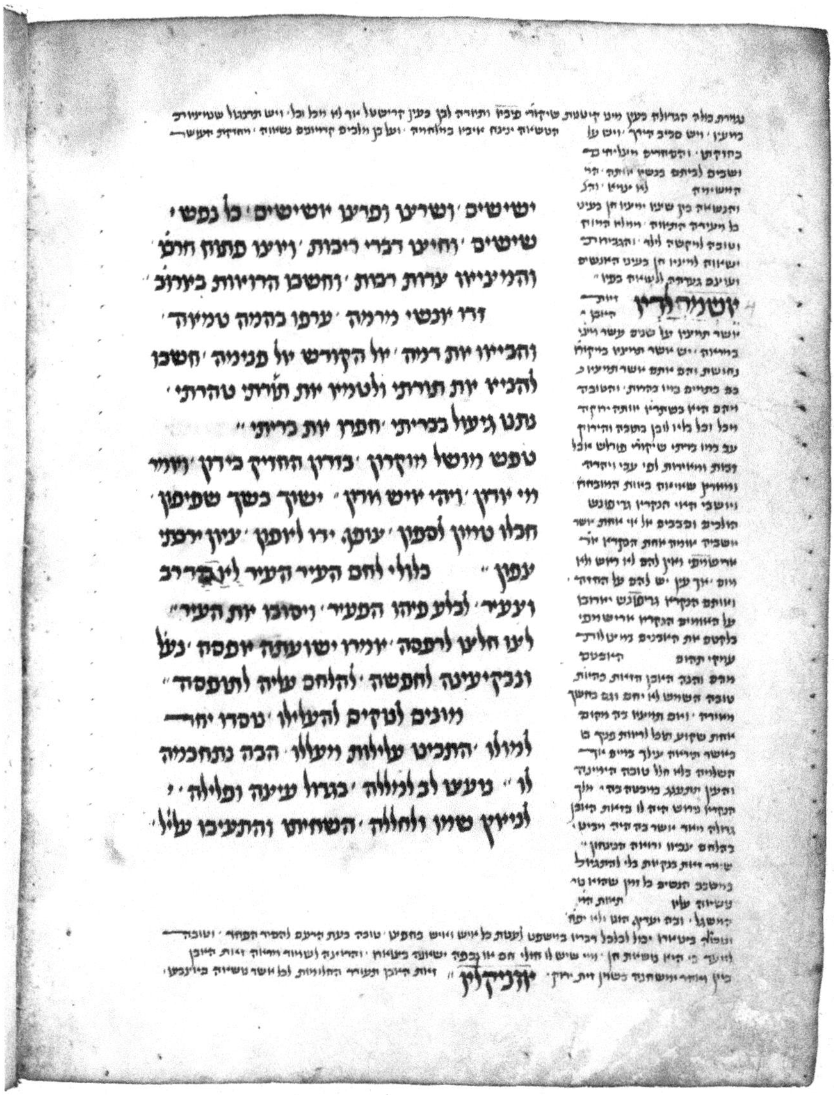

2. fol. 73^v

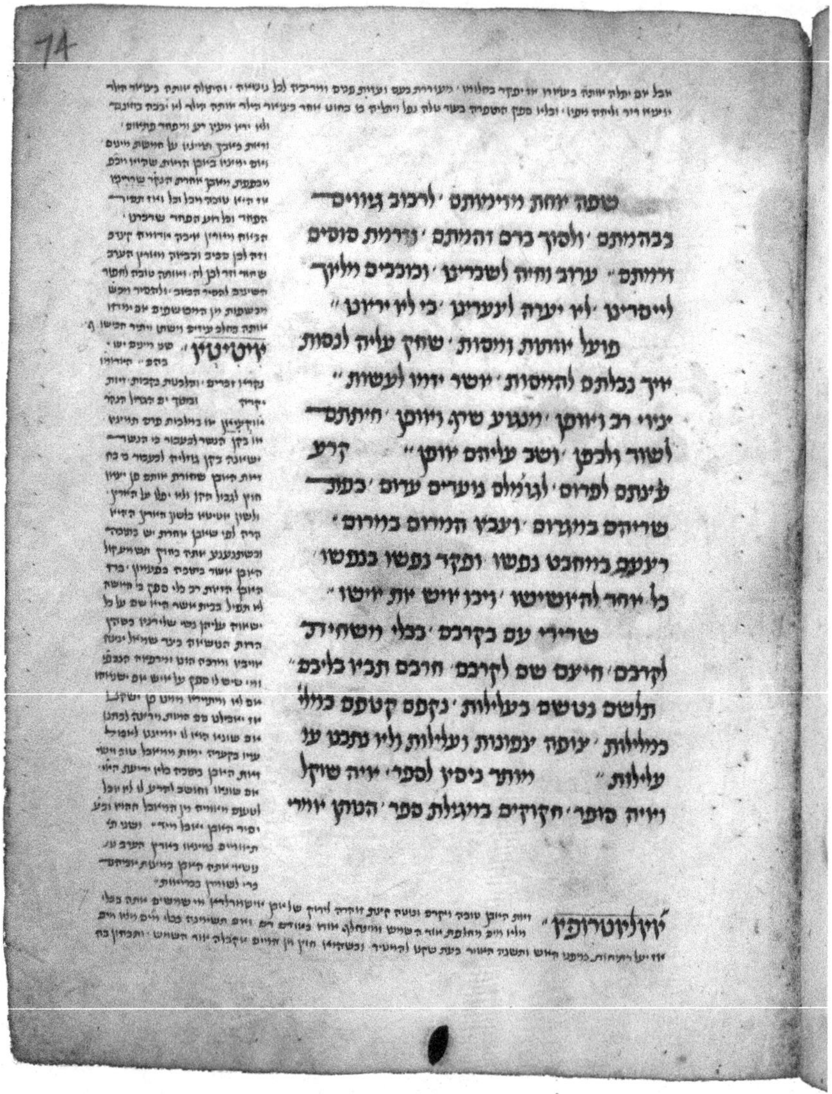

3. fol. 74[r]

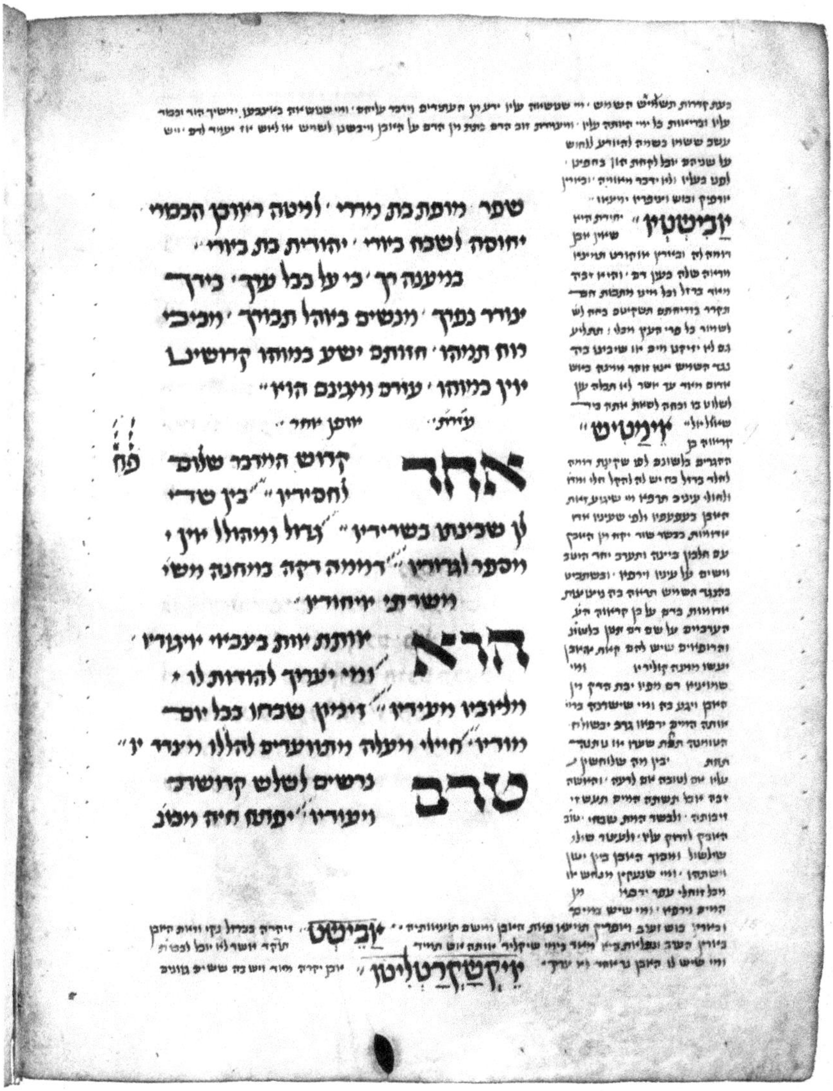

4. fol. 74v

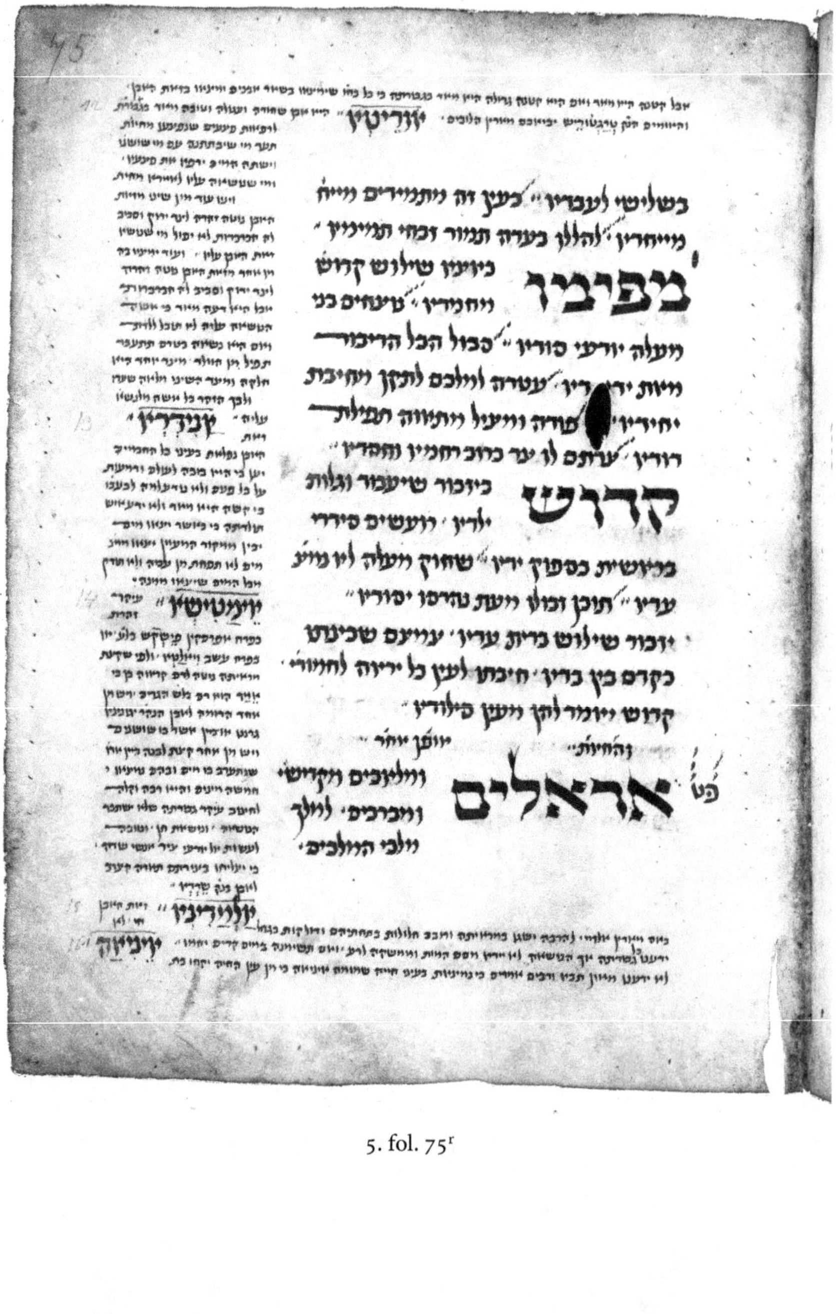

5. fol. 75r

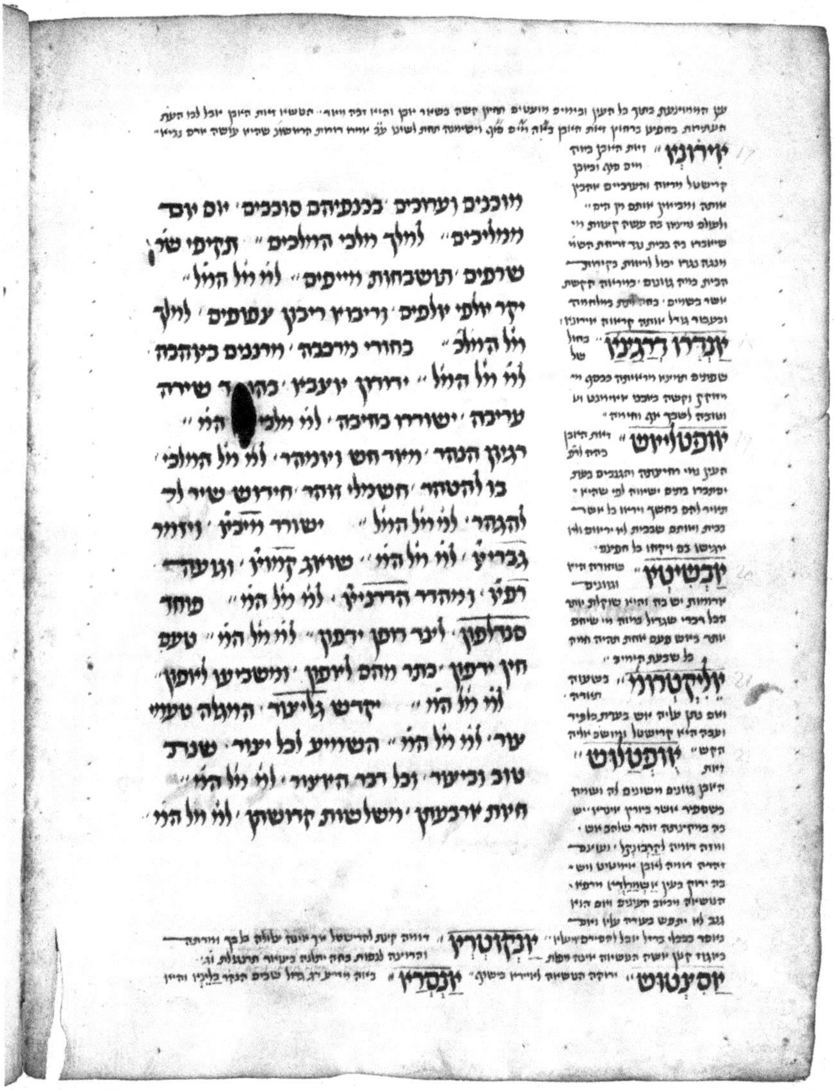

6. fol. 75[v]

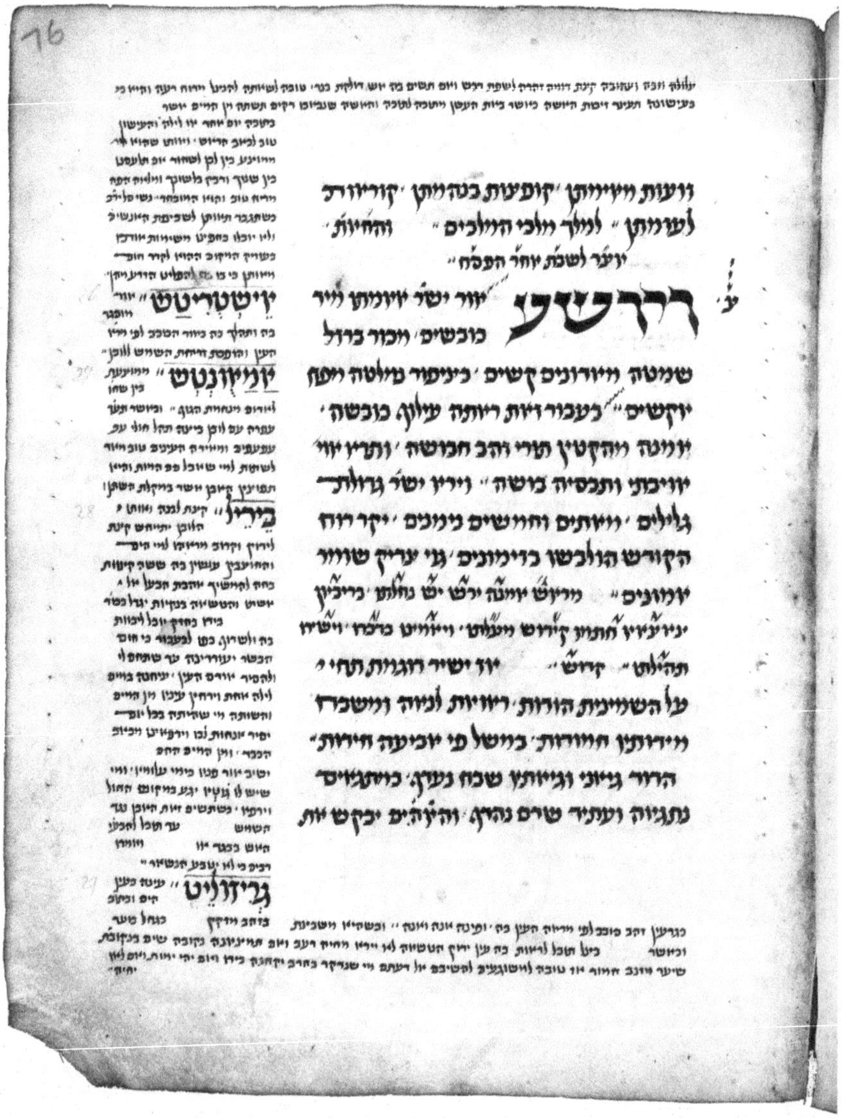

7. fol. 76r

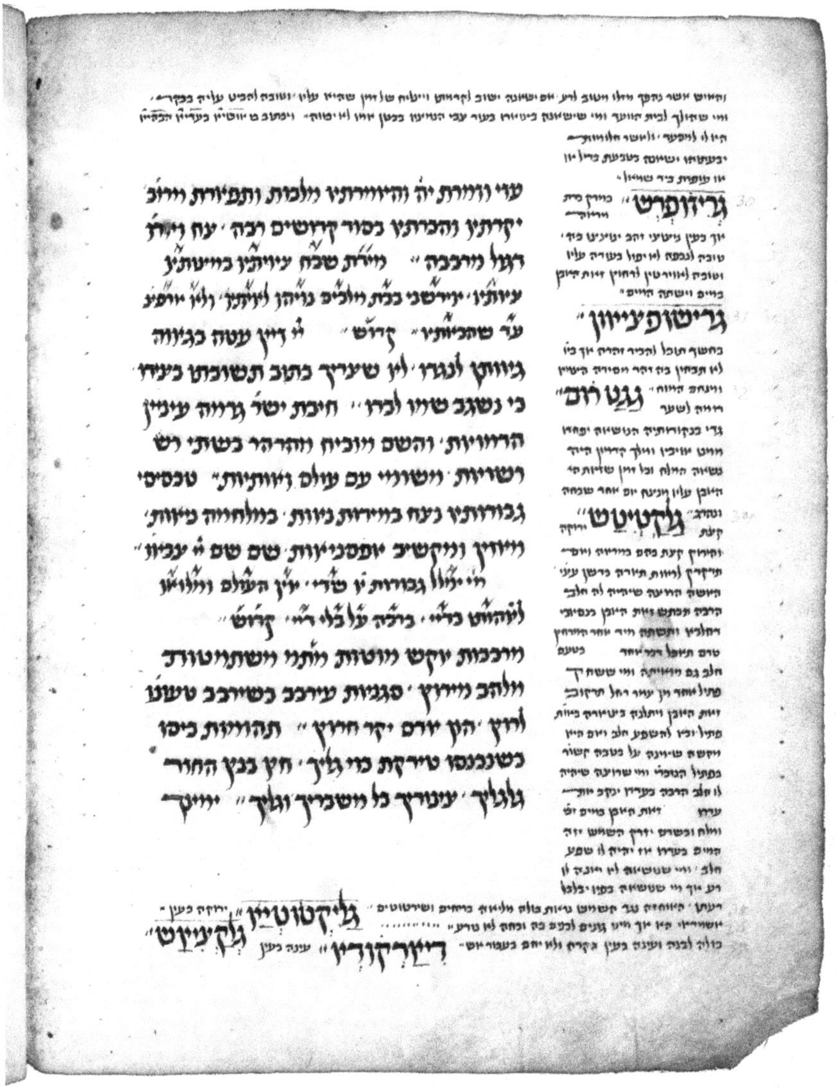

8. fol. 76ᵛ

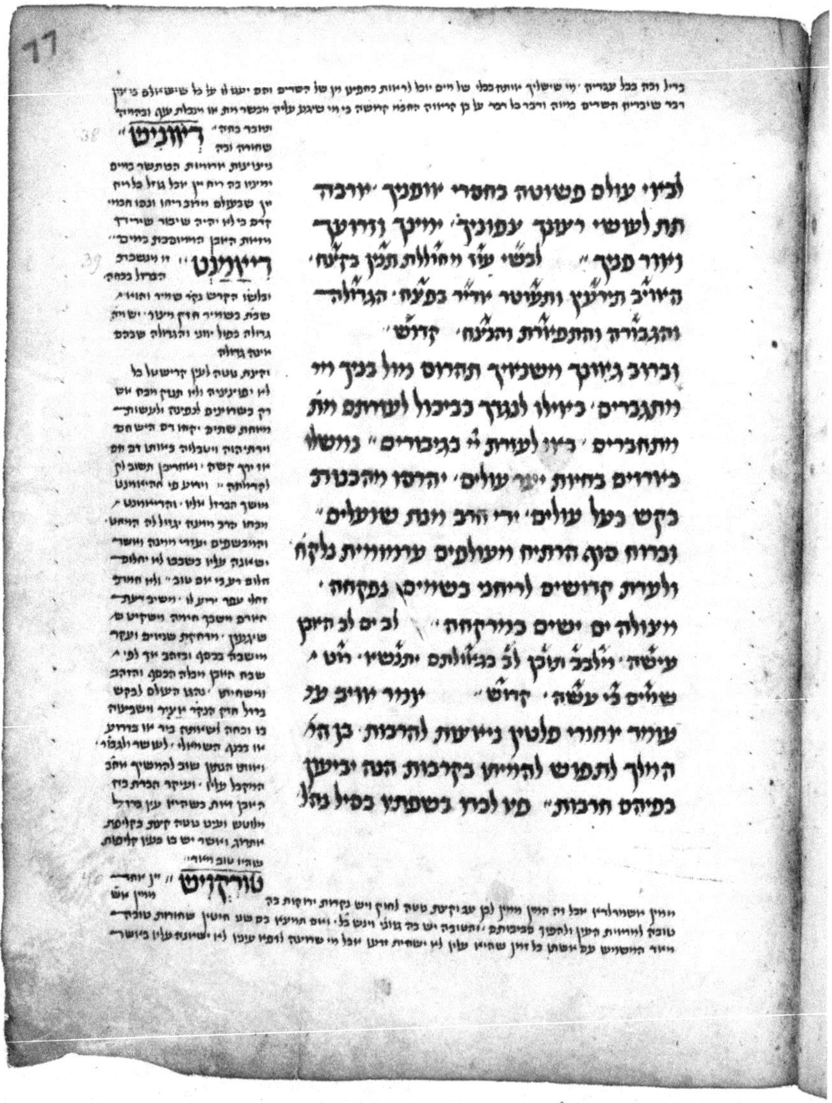

9. fol. 77r

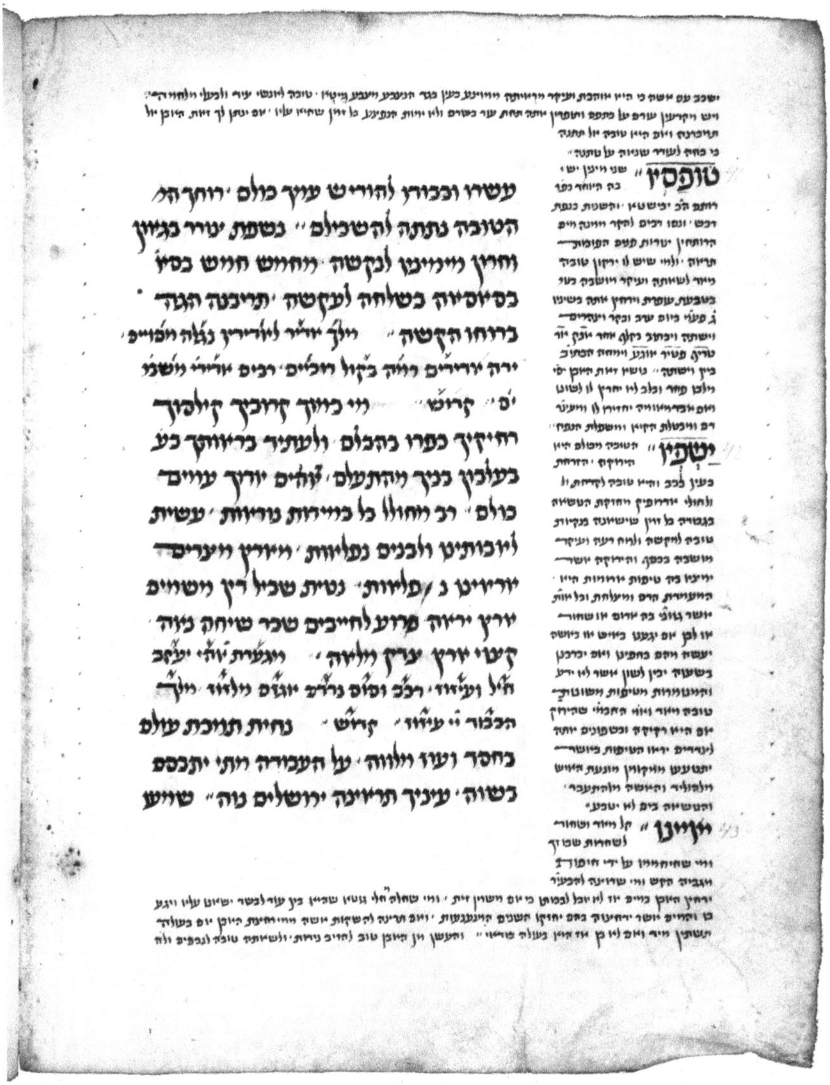

10. fol. 77v

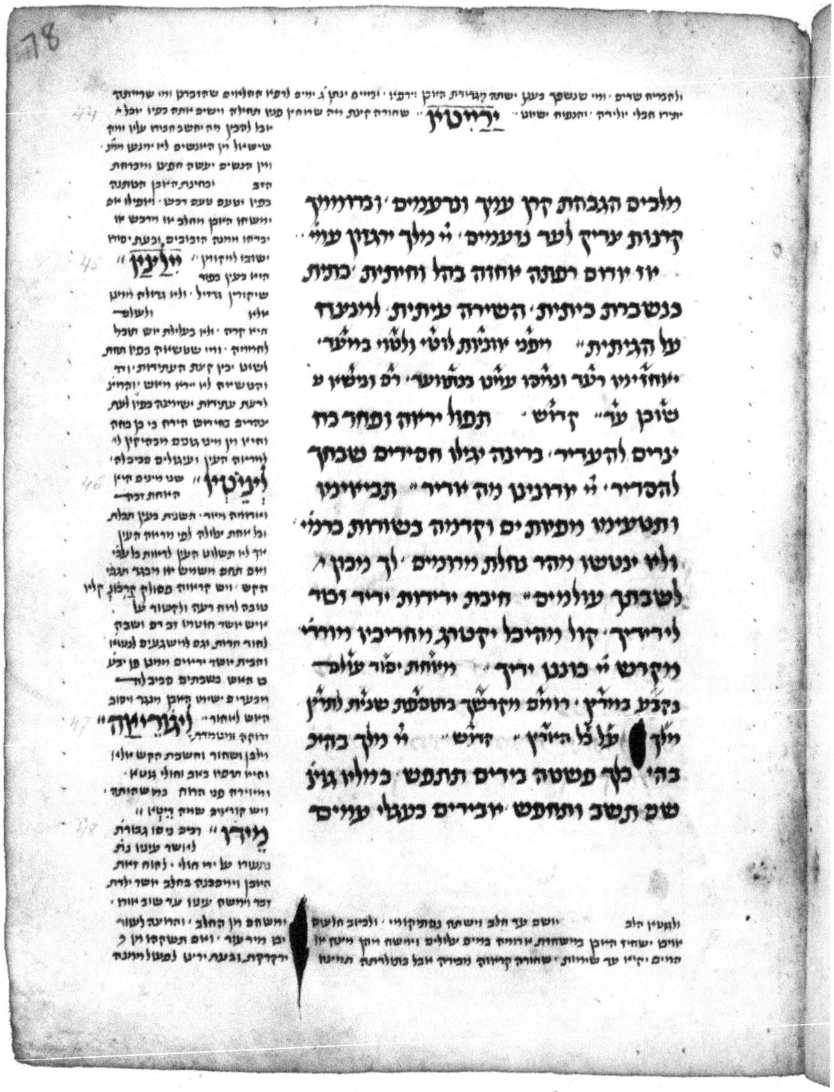

11. fol. 78r

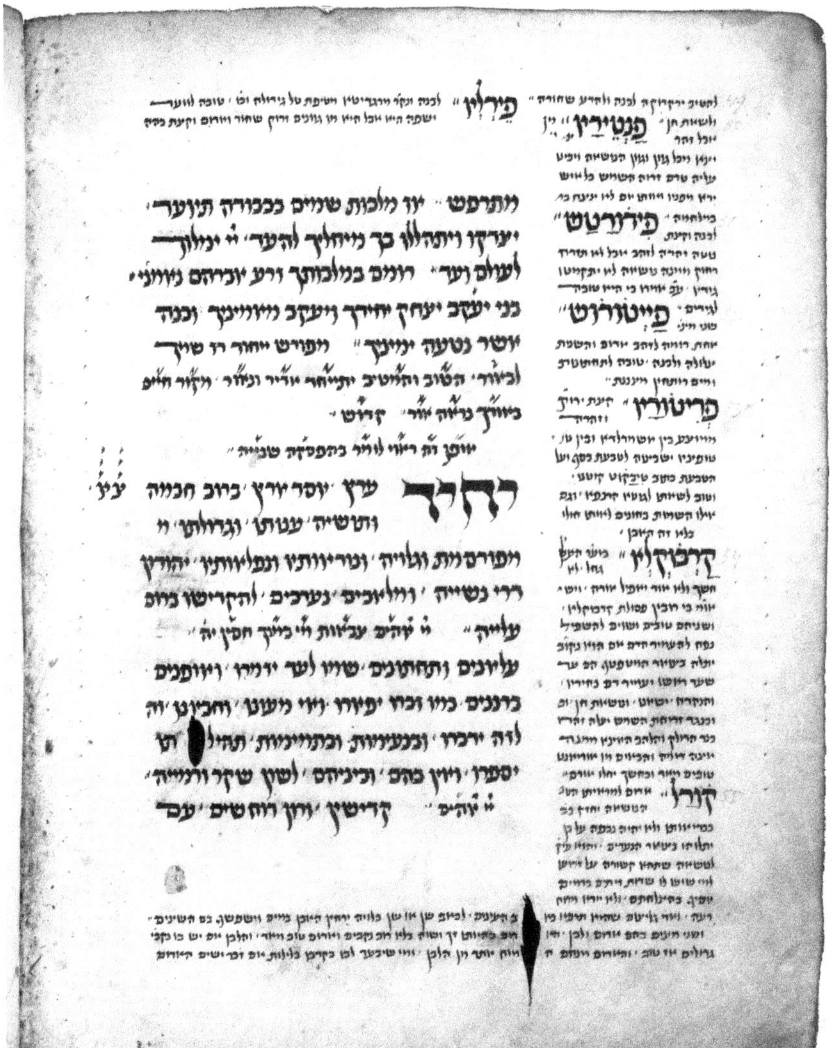

12. fol. 78v

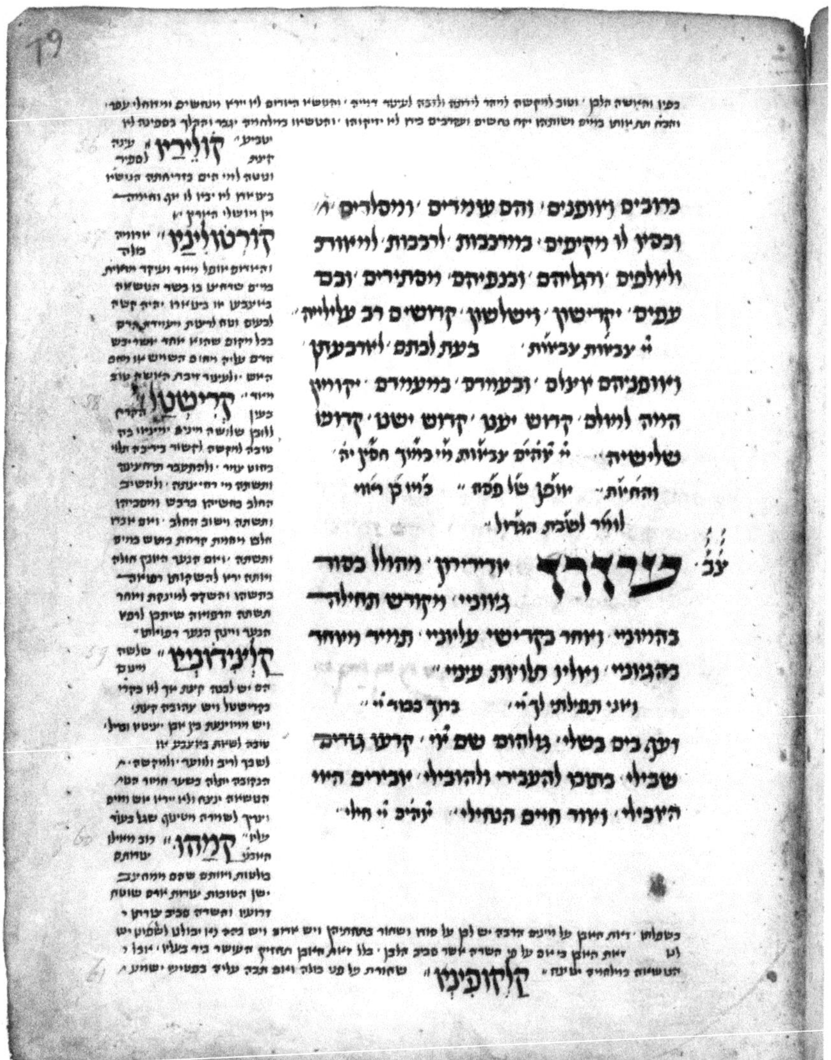

13. fol. 79r

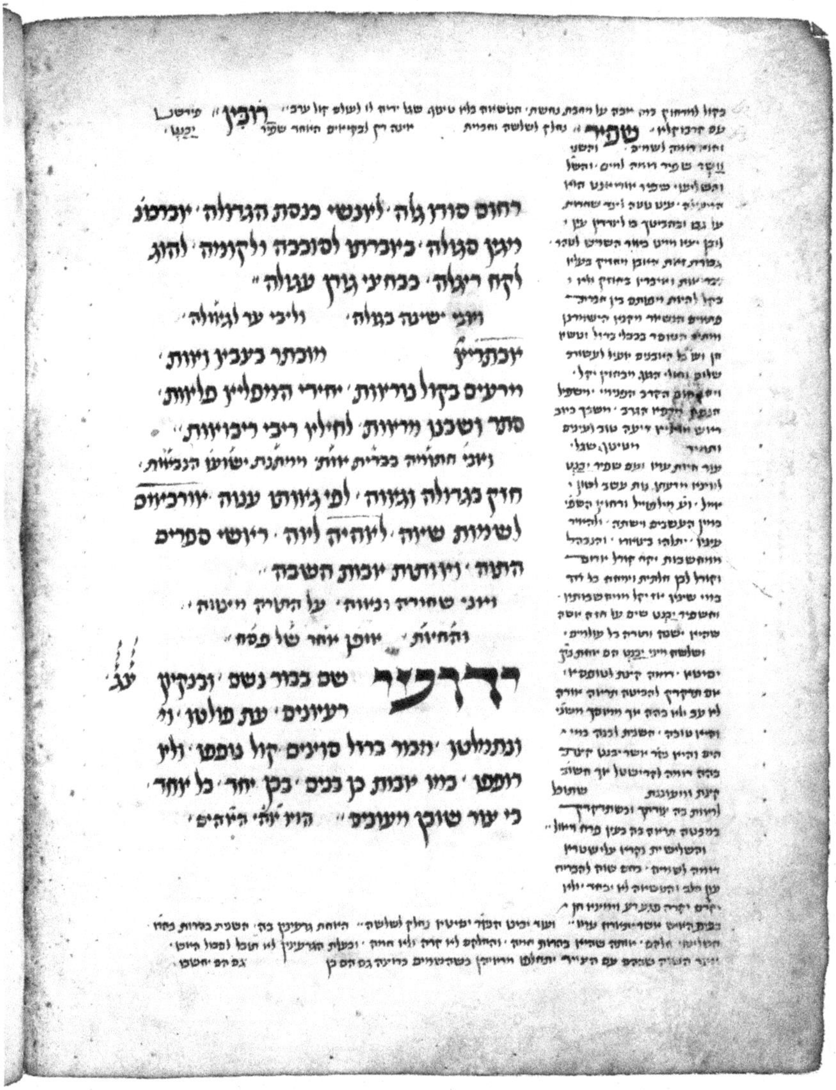

14. fol. 79v

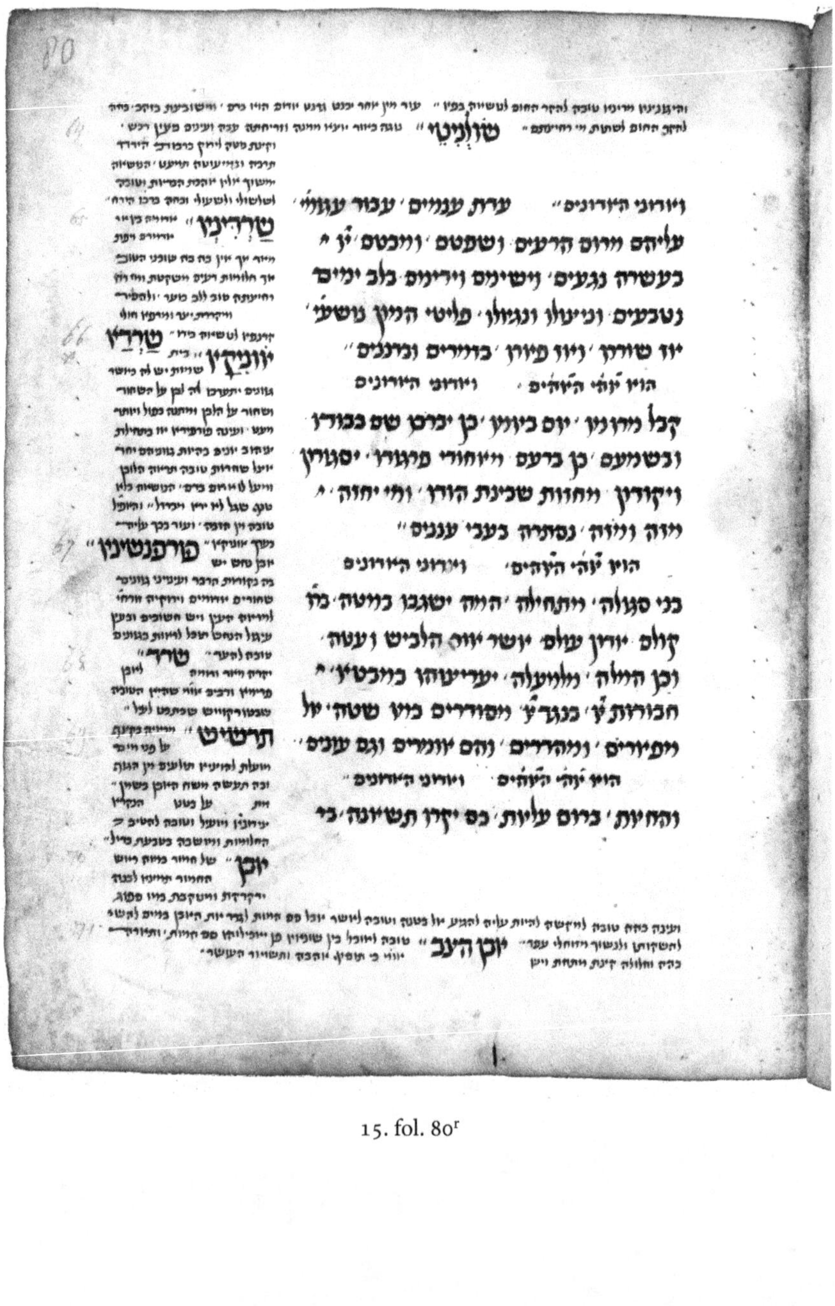

15. fol. 80[r]

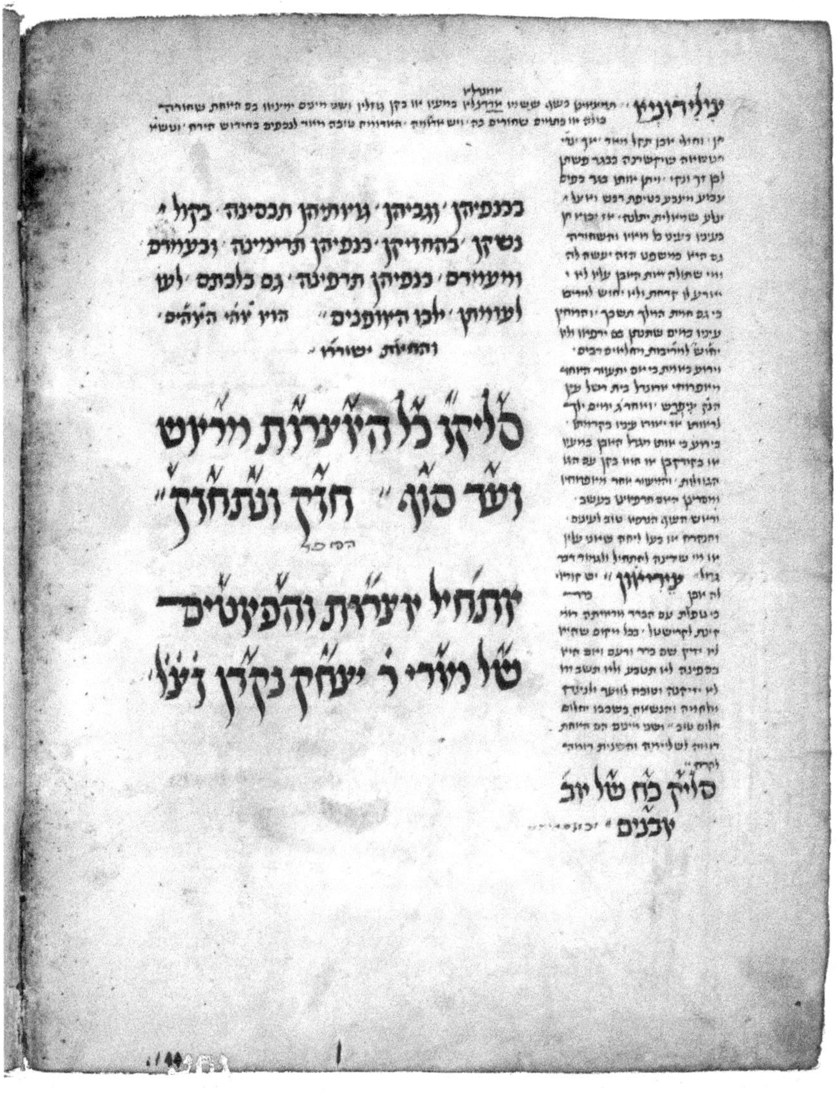

16. fol. 80v

www.ingramcontent.com/pod-product-compliance
Lightning Source LLC
LaVergne TN
LVHW080847300926
849162LV00003B/367